fpa contraceptive handbook

A guide for family planning and other health professionals

Toni Belfield
Director of Information
Family Planning Association

Third edition

Published by the Family Planning Association
2-12 Pentonville Road, London N1 9FP

© Family Planning Association 1999

First edition published 1993
Reprinted 1994 with revisions
Second edition published 1997

British Library Cataloguing in Publication Data
A catalogue record for this book is available from the
British Library.

ISBN 1 899194 76 2

Designed by Andrew Haig & Associates
Geoffrey Haddon, Heleen Franken
Design consultant Peter Gill
Illustrations by Sean MacGarry
Cover photograph by Paul Mattock

Printed in Great Britain by
The College Hill Press Limited

Contents

Acknowledgements   Thank you to the following who gave their time to provide helpful comments and advice: John Guillebaud (Professor of Family Planning and Reproductive Health Care and Medical Director, Margaret Pyke Centre), David Back (Professor of Pharmacology and Therapeutics, University of Liverpool), Dr Connie Smith (Consultant in Family Planning and Reproductive Health Care; Director, Services for Women, Parkside Health NHS Trust; Chair of **fpa**'s Clinical Advisory Committee), Dr Sam Rowlands (GP) and Colin Parker (Managing Director of FP Sales Ltd).

A special thank you to Jane Urwin (**fpa** Medical Information Officer), the CES Helpline Team of Joan Gott, Lynn Hearton and Veronica Smith and to Kate Godwin (**fpa** Publications Manager) for editing the text.

Foreword

This new edition of the **fpa contraceptive handbook** once again provides a clear, concise review of contraceptive practice. It affords comprehensive, useful and well-ordered technical information for those seeking to support women in their choice and use of appropriate contraception. It also helpfully considers the individual and social contexts in which those choices are made. This handbook will be a useful resource both for those with a special interest in contraceptive care, and for the more general reader. It provides accessible and accurate information for primary care, contraceptive clinic practice, and others providing sexual health care. Its contents have been informed by the work of the **fpa** over almost 70 years. Most particularly it has been shaped in response to the questions asked by the public and professionals of the Contraceptive Education Service Helpline provided by the **fpa.**

The place of contraception in the wider picture of sexual health is crucial. This handbook will be a significant contribution to the information available to improve care for all sexual health providers.

Connie Smith
Consultant in Family Planning and Reproductive Health Care; Director, Services for Women, Parkside Health NHS Trust; Chair, Clinical Advisory Committee **fpa**

Introduction

This handbook is intended for family planning professionals and other health professionals who work within the area of reproductive and sexual health. All professionals work within their own professional codes of conduct and these codes govern daily practice.

The handbook aims to provide a convenient and comprehensive guide to contraceptive methods and services. In addition it addresses other areas of reproductive and sexual health such as pre-pregnancy care, sexually transmitted infections and abortion. It is not, and does not set out to be, a comprehensive clinical text book. The handbook is designed to provide quick, easy access to information. Full details about content are given at the beginning of each chapter, and suggested further reading is included at the end of each chapter for those who want more information.

Involving people in the management of their health through the provision of information and the parallel growth of patient and advocacy groups, has resulted in people having access to information from a variety of sources. Some sources are accurate, providing up-to-date and impartial information, but many are not, providing inaccurate, misleading and sometimes sensationalist misinformation.

Knowing about contraception and being able to make informed choices about methods are fundamental issues contributing greatly to the health and well-being of us all. But, how contraception is *considered, discussed* and, most importantly, *delivered* will determine just how well it is accepted *and* used. Recognising that these all interrelate and acknowledging the need to improve the uptake and use of contraceptive methods is as important as recognising that choice of contraception is inextricably linked with emotional and sexual well-being. It is impossible to talk about family planning and contraception without addressing sexuality. Professionals working in these areas need to recognise and acknowledge that because of this, contraception continues to be a source of considerable embarrassment and anxiety for both women and men, and this has implications for its uptake and usage. This embarrassment can have an inhibiting effect on people's willingness to seek information and advice from professionals, and a professional's ability to provide effective care.

Contraception, sexual and reproductive health, more than any other branch of medicine, is an area where a partnership between the public and health professionals is vital. The provision of full, accurate and objective information contributes to that partnership and through such information truly informed choices and decisions can be made.

A final note

This handbook cannot, and is not intended to, replace appropriate training. Family planning and sexual health are not wholly medical issues. The **fpa**'s experience from almost 70 years of working with family planning providers, and of handling over 150,000 enquiries annually from professionals and the public, confirms the need for all those working in the field of family planning and sexual health to have appropriate clinical and non-clinical training. This should involve an awareness of sexuality, an exploration of values and attitudes and the development of communication and active listening skills. Such training will enable professionals to work with women and men of all ages, abilities, cultures, faiths or values and to respond appropriately.

Family planning and sexual health services

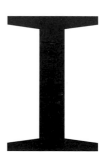

The need for family planning, sexual and reproductive health services

Family planning, sexual and reproductive health are essential parts of preventive health care and an important area of public health. Family planning was defined as an essential component of primary health care in the Alma-Ata Declaration of 1978. This was also a key area in the Department of Health's 1992 health strategy for England, *The Health of the Nation*, which stated:

'Planned parenthood provides benefits for the health of individuals, families and communities. Family planning services aim to promote this by providing access to contraception, sterilisation and advice on unplanned pregnancy. Additionally, education, counselling and health promotion can enable prospective parents to choose healthy lifestyles and increase the chances that their children will be wanted and healthy. Delaying and spacing pregnancies and limiting family size contributes to the physical and mental health of mothers and children and general family well-being.

Purchasers should be aware of the potential of family planning services to improve health by the prevention of unplanned pregnancies and by other health promotion strategies and should work with all appropriate agencies to ensure that services available to local people are complementary and meet identified needs.'

fpa definition of sexual health

Family planning embraces far more than just the methods of contraception; it is part of and includes reproductive health. Family planning aims to enable people to choose whether and when to have children. This includes birth control, planning a baby, timing conception, spacing births and infertility advice and help. Family planning encompasses emotional well-being and affects the individual's enjoyment of his or her own sexuality.

The **fpa** believes that:
'Sexual health is the capacity and freedom to enjoy and express sexuality without fear of exploitation, oppression, physical or emotional harm.'

Sexual health, sexuality and family planning are issues of national concern. They directly affect the health and well-being of present and future generations and must have a place both in public health strategies and in health promotion work. The **fpa** seeks to promote informed choice not only by ensuring that people have access to accurate information, awareness and knowledge of sexual health and family planning, but also by encouraging appropriate social measures, policies and legislation. Those providing family planning services should recognise that an individual's requirements will vary depending on gender, age, class, race, culture or disability, and that equality of opportunity in sexual health and family planning is vital.

Comprehensive and free NHS family planning services

Until the mid-1970s the **fpa** developed and ran well over 1,000 UK family planning clinics. Under the National Health Service Re-organisation Act 1973 (which came into force in 1974) all contraceptive services became free within the National Health Service. As a result the **fpa**'s family planning clinics were incorporated into the NHS. Community family planning clinics are now commissioned by health authorities in England and Wales (health boards in Scotland and Northern Ireland), and provided by community trusts (and a few hospital trusts). In 1975, general practitioners also agreed to provide free family planning services and most GPs now offer contraceptive advice and methods, though not necessarily all methods (eg condoms).

Women and men are free to choose where they go for family planning advice and supplies. This applies to anyone irrespective of age, sex or marital status. Free contraceptive services are available from primary health care professionals (GPs, practice nurses, midwives, health visitors), community family planning clinics, young people's services such as Brook Advisory Centres, in hospitals, through a domiciliary service and many genitourinary medicine (GUM)/sexual health clinics. Private non-profit agencies such as the Marie Stopes clinics and the British Pregnancy Advisory Service (BPAS) will charge a fee.

At present, over 25 per cent of women and men receive family planning advice and methods from health authority community clinics, and over 70 per cent from the primary health care team. Although many people are happy to obtain family planning advice and methods from their primary health care team, services from community-based clinics and domiciliary services or genitourinary medicine clinics are vital for a number of reasons. Most important of these are choice and the recognition that these complement, rather than duplicate, services provided by GPs. NHS Management Executive advice *(Department of Health EL (90) MB 115, June 1990)* determines that family planning should be regarded (and funded) as an 'open access' service. Stated government policy remains that:

'people should be free to choose their source of contraceptive advice and that health authority family planning services complement, rather than duplicate, those which GPs provide. Choice is important to ensure that all those who wish to use this service can do so.'

Choice of family planning services

Evidence shows that there is a relationship between the range of service choices available and the use of contraception – essentially, easier access to services which provide a range of contraceptive choices increases contraceptive uptake and use. There is a complex relationship between quality and accessibility of contraceptive services and method uptake, use and discontinuation. This means that ensuring choice of method and of provider is a crucial element of effective service provision.

Many people are apprehensive about seeking advice and information about family planning. Accessibility, convenience, confidentiality and anonymity are key factors affecting service use. Health professionals can therefore play an important role by providing relevant information and enabling women and men to use family planning services more effectively.

Because family planning embraces more than just the mechanics of contraception, and includes reproductive and sexual health, its wider health role should be reflected in all the services that are offered. The following guidelines are suggested:

Service provision

Family planning provision should include:

▶ a full range of contraceptive methods, including condoms and postcoital contraception
▶ counselling and referral for male and female sterilisation
▶ pregnancy testing, information and counselling for unplanned pregnancy, and referral for abortion
▶ pre-pregnancy advice
▶ advice and help with regard to sexual health and 'safer sex'
▶ help or referral for sexual and relationship problems
▶ well-woman/well-man services
▶ advice, treatment or referral for sexually transmitted infections (STIs), including HIV
▶ advice, help or referral for infertility
▶ advice, help or referral for the menopause and premenstrual tension (PMT)

Service provision should:

▶ be accessible and flexible (location, times of opening)
▶ be appropriately targeted (addressing the sexual and reproductive health care needs of the community)
▶ provide sufficient time for family planning consultations, especially the first and second visits where more time is needed for discussion, and the choosing and teaching of a method
▶ be effective (designed, developed and delivered on the basis of local needs assessment)
▶ be efficient and of good quality (audited services)

▶ be known about (good advertising within and outside the service)

▶ provide an assurance of confidentiality in visits, communications and record keeping

▶ provide a choice (where possible) of male or female doctor

▶ have appropriate referral mechanisms

Training

▶ ensure all staff (including reception and clerical staff) are appropriately trained and supported by updating of knowledge and skills

▶ recognise the different professional roles and maximise this potential

Information

▶ always provide standardised, complete, up-to-date and impartial information, ie the information that *you* yourself would expect to receive

▶ use suitable up-to-date language that both enables and informs, eg talk about IUDs, progestogen-only pills, natural family planning and postcoital (or emergency) contraception; do not talk about coils, mini-pills, rhythm methods or morning-after contraception

▶ always discuss risks, benefits and uncertainties

▶ recognise that people are not always comfortable and may not feel able to ask questions

▶ check out information needs of clients

▶ always provide appropriate and accessible written information that backs up and reinforces any verbal advice

▶ provide interpreting services for those whose first language is not English

▶ recognise the need for cultural sensitivity

▶ provide information about services so people know about them

Research and study over the years have shown that family planning clinics and general practices may be perceived differently, and that some women use both types of service for different purposes. Issues such as the availability of more specialist/expert help, more time, availability of female staff and wider choice of method have been identified as advantages of community clinic provision. Services through general practice are seen as offering more continuity of care and easier availability and anonymity (in that other people attending the surgery may not know the reason for the visit).

Such knowledge highlights the importance of ensuring that all women and men can easily gain access to a choice of contraceptive providers.

NHS community family planning clinics

Most community family planning clinics are provided by community NHS trusts. In a few areas it is the hospital trust that provides clinic services. Some health authorities also purchase services from providers such as Brook Advisory Centres. The characteristics of clinic services include:

► staff with appropriate family planning training
► a full range of contraceptive methods is usually available (newer methods such as implants and intrauterine systems may not be so widely available)
► information, advice and counselling on a wide range of sexual and reproductive health issues
► specialist services for young people
► easily available emergency contraception
► provision of training for doctors and nurses in family planning (not all)
► undertaking of research – clinical and psychosocial (not all)

Procedures at clinics

At the first visit to a family planning clinic the client's name, address and age are noted as are the name and address of their GP. Permission should always be sought at this stage as to whether or not a GP may be contacted, and how a client can be contacted by the clinic. Confidentiality should be ensured in visits, communications and in record keeping. This is vital for all clients, but especially teenagers.

A physical examination (in the absence of a problem or a request) is *not* required at a first visit unless a diaphragm, cap, IUD or intrauterine system (IUS) is to be used. Clients are generally seen by a nurse or a doctor.

Contraceptive supplies are provided at the clinic. If the client's GP is to be informed about any chosen method it should be stressed that this will only be with the person's permission. Cervical cytology results are also sent to a client's GP, with permission only.

Primary health care team family planning provision

Most GPs provide a contraceptive service. A person may see their own GP or choose to find another GP who offers a family planning service without a referral. The primary health care team also includes the practice nurse, midwife and health visitor. It may also include the school nurse. Currently there is no mandatory requirement for GPs or nurses to have post-qualification training in family planning. They may have varying levels of training and experience in family planning.

Doctors can arrange for clients/patients to go elsewhere (eg to a community family planning clinic or hospital department) for any family planning service which they may not give; for example, not all may provide diaphragms, caps, IUDs, the IUS or implants. Male and female condoms are often not available from GPs.

Family planning supplies are dispensed free of charge on a prescription with the exception of condoms. Prescriptions are dispensed by a community pharmacist in most cases – or by a dispenser in a dispensing practice.

Nurses

Research shows consistent satisfaction with nurses as providers of contraceptive advice and services. Yet practice nurses are often under-utilised. With appropriate training, agreed protocols and access to medical support, family planning nurses can provide a quality service that is 'user friendly' and also cost-effective to the purchaser. Nurse prescribing has now been under discussion for well over 20 years. The Medicinal Products: Prescribing by Nurses Act (1992) permits registered nurses, health visitors and midwives to prescribe from a limited formulary of products. The Act gives the Secretary of State the power to limit the formulary and to set categories.

Because it was felt that too little was known to extend nurse prescribing, the Department of Health (DH), set up a pilot programme in October 1994. This aims to obtain information on the impact of nurse prescribing on quality of care, timesaving and cost benefit. The scheme, initially in eight sites, has now been extended. However, it does not include family planning nurses, nor does the formulary include contraception despite the fact that this area is ideal for inclusion. While nurse prescribing in family planning is currently unlawful, nurse issuing is commonplace, and has the support of the United Kingdom Central Council (UKCC), the RCN and the Medical Defence Union (MDU). Protocol-led services have been set up by organisations such as Brook and the Margaret Pyke Centre in London. The Crown Report 1998, *The Review of Prescribing, Supply and Administration of Medicines: Report on Supply and Administration of Medicines under Group Protocols* recognises the need for flexibility in making greater use of the skills and experience of the various professionals working in primary care. This Report makes recommendations about current and future practice under group protocols, widening the availability of licensed drugs.

Domiciliary family planning

Domiciliary family planning services are provided in some areas of the UK and involve a doctor or nurse making a home visit. Alternatively, they may accompany the client if they are unable to go on their own to a community clinic or to a GP for advice and help on contraception. A member of the primary health care team can arrange this.

Genitourinary medicine (GUM) clinics/sexual health clinics

Many genitourinary medicine (GUM) clinics now provide contraceptive services, especially emergency contraception. These clinics are referred to by various names: *STD clinics, Special clinics, VD clinics, GU* or *GUM clinics.* Some just have names (eg Lydia) which seemingly have no connection with sexually transmitted infections. The term *sexual health clinic/service* is being promoted, recognising the need to provide a more holistic sexual and reproductive health service.

Young people

Specialist contraceptive, sexual and reproductive health care services for young people are now widely available in most health authorities as a result of *The Health of the Nation* initiatives. These provide services that are free, confidential, accessible and appropriate and include the wider education, social information, counselling and health care needs of young people.

See also Brook Advisory Centres, page 180.

Other family planning services

There are various non-NHS family planning clinics in the UK. Some are private and others are charitable. Some operate on the basis of contractual arrangements with the NHS.

Some offer a fee-paying service in various parts of the country, such as the British Pregnancy Advisory Service, the Marie Stopes clinics (Marie Stopes International).

The **fpa**, through the Contraceptive Education Service (CES), can provide detailed information on *all* contraceptive methods, family planning clinic services and sexual and reproductive services in the UK (see 'fpa services', page 213). Family planning and health professionals may contact the **fpa** direct or refer enquirers to the **fpa** for information.

Information about family planning services can also be obtained from:

- ▶ the local health authority or health board
- ▶ local health centre/hospital
- ▶ GP, practice nurse, midwife, health visitor, school nurse
- ▶ post office/public library
- ▶ telephone directory, local directory
- ▶ local information centres or health lines

Family planning organisations

The UK Family Planning Association (fpa)

The **fpa** is the leading UK voluntary organisation combining sexual health and family planning. Founded in 1930, the **fpa** has a unique and outstanding reputation, based on pioneering work. Its success in winning the right to family planning and contraception, thus relieving the suffering, ill health and poverty caused by frequent childbearing, is one of the most notable contributions to family life this century. It became a charity in 1962.

After the transfer of its clinics to the NHS in 1974 (see page 11) the **fpa** shifted its focus from direct service provision. Its primary aim is:

'To advance the sexual health and reproductive rights and choices of all people throughout the UK.'

It achieves this through a range of national activities including the Contraceptive Education Service (CES), publications for the public and professionals, research and policy work, consultancy, press and publicity, and practice development, education and training work with professionals.

Through CES, the **fpa** provides full information on all aspects of family planning, contraceptive methods, and sexual and reproductive health, including service provision within the UK. The **fpa** also produces a full range of CES leaflets for the general public on all the different contraceptive methods, and a quarterly publication – the *Contraceptive Education Bulletin* – for professionals (for further information, see '**fpa** services', page 213).

The **fpa** has centres in London, Cardiff, Bangor, Belfast, Derry and Glasgow.

Equality of opportunity in sexual health and family planning is vital. The **fpa** recognises that needs may vary depending on gender, age, class, race, culture, sexual orientation, and mental and physical disability.

Faculty of Family Planning and Reproductive Health Care (FFPRHC) of the Royal College of Obstetricians and Gynaecologists (RCOG)

The Faculty of Family Planning and Reproductive Health Care was established in 1993.

The FFPRHC's aims are to:

▶ give academic status to the discipline of family planning and reproductive health care and recognise the expertise within it
▶ maintain and develop standards of care and training and ensure that a high quality of practice is maintained by all providers of family planning and reproductive health care
▶ promote the effective interaction of reproductive health care with related disciplines
▶ gather, collate and provide information in support of basic and continuing education in the discipline
▶ advance medical knowledge in the discipline and encourage audit and research
▶ support and represent those working in the discipline at regional, national and international levels

The FFPRHC awards two qualifications: membership (MFFP) and Diploma (DFFP). Qualification for the DFFP is through practical and theoretical training. Entry to membership is by examination. Additional certification (Letters of Competence) is provided for intrauterine techniques, subdermal implants and postgraduate education. Additional certification will also include other specialist areas in the future as innovative contraceptive products become available.

The FFPRHC has affiliated groups of family planning doctors throughout the UK and in the Republic of Ireland. The Faculty provides conferences and lectures, and publishes the quarterly *British Journal of Family Planning*. The work of the Faculty's Clinical Effectiveness Committee includes the development of short evidence-based guidelines for members, and responding to individual members' enquiries about contraceptive and reproductive health care provision. The database established by the former National Co-ordinating Unit for Clinical Audit in Family Planning has been transferred to the Faculty's London offices.

National Association of Nurses for Contraception and Sexual Health (NANCSH)

The National Association of Family Planning Nurses (NAFPN) became NANCSH in 1995. Membership of NANCSH is open to all registered nurses, midwives and health visitors who hold a recognised family planning qualification. Associate membership is open to those who have an interest or involvement in family planning. NANCSH's aims are:

▶ the advancement of education by the promotion of interest in and the increased knowledge of all matters appertaining to male and female sexual and reproductive health
▶ to facilitate the study and exchange of information and ideas on contraception and sexual health by seminars, workshops, discussions, meetings and exhibitions
▶ to promote and maintain high standards of education and training in patient care and encourage audit and research
▶ to promote a holistic approach to sexual health education

NANCSH publishes the *NANCSH Journal.*

Royal College of Nursing (RCN) Family Planning Forum

This is one of a number of special interest groups of the Royal College of Nursing. Membership is free to all registered nurses, midwives and health visitors who are RCN members. Its main objectives are to:

- ▶ establish a corporate identity for RCN members engaged in the specialty of family planning nursing
- ▶ increase knowledge and skills in family planning
- ▶ act as a resource to the RCN

The Scottish Society for Family Planning Nurses

This Association represents the interests of nurses working in family planning in Scotland.

The Northern Ireland Association of Family Planning Nurses

This Association represents the interests of nurses working in family planning in Northern Ireland.

Family planning and the pharmacist

Pharmacists have a fund of knowledge that is valuable to family planning and health professionals. Pharmacists often receive more direct feedback from patients than other health professionals especially about factors such as compliance and palatability of medicines. Pharmacists often see people with initial concerns or worries and are therefore in a good position to refer.

Pharmacists are fully involved in the wider role of health promotion in the everyday setting of a community pharmacy or hospital. They can advise and supply certain contraceptive methods that do not require a prescription as well as dispensing contraception on prescription. Recommendations in the Crown Report (see page 17) refer also to pharmacists. They are therefore in constant contact with people who may seek advice about contraception and related areas. Because pharmacists are not perceived as 'authoritarian' medical figures and are easily accessible in pharmacies, they have an invaluable role in providing information about family planning and sexual health and in enabling women and men to seek further help effectively from health and medical professionals. Pharmacists' knowledge of medical matters, and specifically of drugs and drug interactions, make them an important part of the health care team today.

About six million people visit a pharmacy every day in the UK. Recognising the potential to reach the public, the Pharmacy Healthcare Scheme was set up in 1986 to promote comprehensive health care information through all UK pharmacies. Contraception and sexual health care issues feature regularly. The scheme is run by the Royal Pharmaceutical Society of Great Britain.

Further reading

Books

*The economics of family planning services –
a report prepared for the Contraceptive Alliance*
McGuire A and Hughes D
fpa, 1995

The fight for family planning
Leathard A
Macmillan Press, 1980

*It's more than weight and blood pressure ...
the enhanced role of the family planning nurse*
Brook Advisory Centres, 1996

Report

*A report on the supply and administration of medicines
under group protocols (Chairman, Dr June Crown)*
Prescribing, Supply and Administration of Medicines
Review Team
Department of Health, 1998

Articles

'Nurse only family planning clinics'
Ross G
British Journal of Family Planning, 21, 1996, 142-144

'Family planning provision in genitourinary medicine
clinics: a quiet revolution'
Walsh J
British Journal of Family Planning, 22, 1996, 27-30

'Destigmatising sexual health clinics'
Greenhouse P
British Journal of Sexual Medicine, 23, 1996, 13-16

'Pharmacists as counsellors?'
Rees J A
Pharmaceutical Journal, 257, 1996, 200

Conception

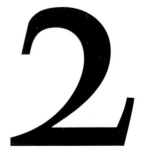

The male

Sperm production

Sperm are produced in the seminiferous tubules within the testes. They then move into the epididymis where they mature and develop. From production to maturity takes about three months and is a continual process. Mature sperm pass through the vasa deferentia to be stored in the seminal vesicles near the prostate gland. When a man is sexually excited and has an erection, the stored sperm enter the urethra where secretions from the prostate are added. This fluid is the semen and it is expelled by contractions of the penis during ejaculation. A single normal semen specimen can contain 300 million sperm per cubic millimetre. Each one is 1/500 inch in length. Sperm survival in the female reproductive tract is regarded to be in the region of three to seven days, with three to five being optimum for fertilisation. Semen analysis will consider number, motility and morphology.

The female

Ovulation

A woman's menstrual cycle begins with the onset of the menstrual period. This cycle is controlled by the pituitary hormones – follicle stimulating hormone (FSH) and luteinising hormone (LH) – and the ovarian hormones oestrogen and progesterone. The pituitary hormones trigger follicle development where one of the eggs within the ovary matures and, about 12-16 days before the beginning of her *next* period, the mature egg is released from the ovary. The egg enters the funnel-shaped end of the fallopian tube and is transported down the fallopian tube by contractions of the tube and by movement of cilia lining the tube. Each egg measures about 1/175 of an inch and is about the size of a full stop. Egg survival is about 12-24 hours.

Passage of sperm/cervical mucus

Once in the woman's vagina, the sperm enter the womb through the cervix by passing through the cervical mucus. Cervical mucus plays a vital role in reproduction. Its most important function is to control the transport of sperm from the vagina to the fallopian tube so that fertilisation can occur. When the woman is in the fertile period of her menstrual cycle (around ovulation) 'fertile' cervical mucus is produced which is thin, stretchy and watery; this contains channels that allow sperm to pass into the womb where they swim up to the fallopian tubes. At other times in the cycle, the cervical mucus – 'infertile' mucus – is less easily penetrated: it is thick and impenetrable which inhibits the movement of sperm.

Fertilisation

Fertilisation usually takes place in the fallopian tube. The fertilised egg then travels down to the womb, where under the influence of oestrogen the lining has thickened ready to receive it. The fertilised egg, dividing all the time, begins to implant in the endometrium about five to seven days after ovulation.

Implantation

The implanted early embryo produces a hormone, human chorionic gonadotrophin (hCG), which enters the bloodstream and reaches the ovary where it acts to maintain the corpus luteum. The corpus luteum produces the hormone progesterone which sustains the pregnancy. Not all eggs that are released are fertilised, and of those that are, many do not implant, or fail to develop properly and to establish pregnancy. Because of these factors, medical and legal opinion considers that pregnancy does not begin until implantation.

Contraception

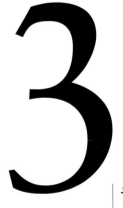

3

General introduction

Contraception involves an interruption in the normal physiological events leading to conception. This is achieved by control of ovulation or by using methods that stop fertilisation by preventing the egg and the sperm meeting. There are many methods available.

Unreliable methods and popular fallacies

There is some truth in the statement that any method is better than none. Probably the most commonly used (but not well-documented) is coitus interruptus or 'withdrawal' (often described as 'being careful'). This method is unreliable because ejaculation can be difficult to control and some sperm may be released before the penis is withdrawn. Those using this method should be given information about other more effective methods. No-one however should be discouraged from using any method if it works for them and they choose not to use another.

Myths

There are many myths about contraception which are inaccurate. Whatever people say, the facts are that:

▶ pregnancy can occur if the woman does not have an orgasm, and intercourse in any position can result in pregnancy
▶ pregnancy can follow the first intercourse, can occur without full penetration, and occasionally results when intercourse takes place during the woman's period (this will relate to a woman's menstrual cycle length)
▶ douching is useless as a contraceptive measure and persistent douching may damage the vaginal mucosa and cause other problems such as infection
▶ pregnancy can occur just after a woman's period

Many people are not sure how their bodies work and may need help in understanding issues around conception and contraception. Health professionals are in an ideal position to provide accurate information and help.

Methods available

Regular methods
- combined oral contraceptive (COC)
- progestogen-only pill (POP)
- contraceptive implants
- the intrauterine system (IUS)
- injectable contraception
- intrauterine contraceptive device (IUD)
- female barrier methods: diaphragm or cap and spermicide, and female condoms
- male condoms
- spermicides
- natural family planning/fertility awareness
- male and female sterilisation

Emergency methods (postcoital contraception)
- hormonal methods
- IUD method

Efficacy of contraceptive methods

See Table 1 for the efficacy of the different methods.

The **fpa** produces Contraceptive Education Service (CES) leaflets for the general public on *all* the methods of contraception (see '**fpa** services', page 213).

Review of the scientific literature reveals a wide range of data about the efficacy of contraceptive methods. Data varies between studies, between countries and between providers. As a result, health professionals and users are understandably confused as to how effective individual methods really are.

Some of the reasons for the lack of comparative data in research around contraceptive efficacy are:

- type of study/study design
- method of data collection
- method of data analysis
- patient characteristics (age, parity, spacers, completed family, etc)
- loss to follow-up

▶ acceptability of product

▶ quality of teaching by health professional/provider

Contraceptive failure rates are significantly higher 'in real life' (user-failure) than in clinical trials which are looking to get information about method failure. User-failure relates to where pregnancy has occurred due to the incorrect use or non-use of a method on one or more occasions. Method-failure relates to where pregnancy has occurred despite the method being used absolutely correctly (or fitted correctly in the case of IUDs, IUS and implants) and consistently for every act of intercourse. For user-dependent methods such as oral contraceptives, male and female barrier methods and natural family planning, failure rates are higher than average within the first 12 months (the 'learning curve') of use. Unintended pregnancy is also more likely to happen when experience of, or anxiety about, side-effects leads to incorrect use or inconsistent use of methods.

Increasing user-effectiveness depends on:

▶ ensuring that women and men know that it is important to use their method correctly and consistently
▶ teaching how to use the method correctly
▶ recognising the difference between what is taught and what is learnt
▶ good initial teaching by going through the method in a 'one to one' situation
▶ providing written information to 'back-up verbal advice'
▶ checking out what has been learnt
▶ providing telephone helplines, or other back-up or referral if more information is needed
▶ encouraging disclosure of any problems, perceptions or anxieties
▶ discussing risks *and* benefits and any uncertainties
▶ advising on the availability and use of 'back-up' methods and of emergency contraception

Table 1 Efficacy of contraceptive methods

% per 100 women per year

Methods that have no 'user' failure	
Injectable contraception	over 99% effective
Implants	over 99% effective in first year (over 98% per year over five years)
Intrauterine system (IUS)	over 99% effective
Intrauterine device (IUD)	98-over 99% effective (depending on IUD type)
Female sterilisation	over 99% effective 1 in 200 lifetime failure rate
Male sterilisation (vasectomy)	over 99% effective 1 in 2000 lifetime failure rate
Methods that have 'user' failure	
Combined oral contraceptive	over 99% effective
Progestogen-only oral contraceptive	up to 99% effective
Male condom	up to 98% effective
Female condom	up to 95% effective
Diaphragm or cap + spermicide	up to 96% effective
Natural family planning: ► combining two or more fertility indicators ► new technologies (Persona)	up to 98% effective up to 94% effective

Note

Efficacy rates of methods with 'user' failure reflect use when used absolutely correctly and consistently. Where methods are used less well, lower efficacy will be seen.

Where contraceptives work

Female

1 Combined pill
▶ prevents ovulation
▶ affects cervical mucus
▶ suppresses the endometrium

2 IUD
▶ prevents sperm reaching the egg

2 IUS
▶ affects cervical mucus
▶ suppresses the endometrium
▶ some effect on ovulation

3 Injectables
▶ prevents ovulation

3 Implants
▶ affects cervical mucus
▶ affects ovulation

4 Sterilisation
▶ prevents egg reaching the womb

5 Diaphragm and cap + spermicide, female condom
▶ prevents sperm reaching the egg

6 Progestogen-only pill
▶ effect mainly on cervical mucus

Natural methods
▶ identifying fertile and infertile times in the menstrual cycle

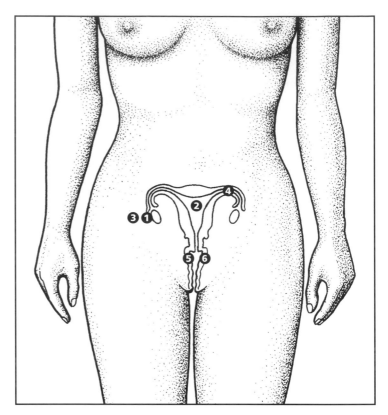

Male

1 Vasectomy
▶ prevents sperm release

2 Male condom
▶ prevents sperm reaching the egg

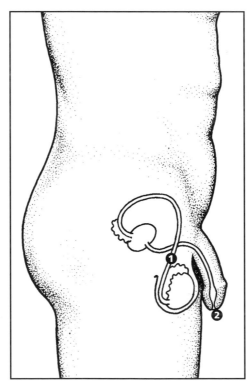

Use of contraceptive methods is also influenced by:

▶ perceptions of how easy it is to use the method correctly and consistently
▶ the way in which method characteristics and method use are portrayed by health professionals
▶ whether the method provided is the method the individual intended to use
▶ the perceived quality of contraceptive services
▶ the perceived effectiveness of client/professional communication
▶ the duration of effect/how often the client has to attend for follow-up

Providing and supporting contraceptive choices depends on:

▶ finding out which method, if any, the individual has in mind
▶ establishing how this choice was made, how well-informed it is, and what underlying needs, priorities and concerns it reflects
▶ supporting informed choice by providing information, increasing motivation and confidence, and offering practical solutions to difficulties
▶ providing opportunities at regular intervals to check knowledge and to discuss concerns
▶ offering opportunities to reconsider contraceptive choices

All of these recognise that contraceptive needs and expectations are influenced by many factors. These include current life-stage and circumstances, motivation for using contraception, and perceptions and beliefs. The methods chosen reflect how people feel about their sexuality and sexual identity, which are further related to feelings of self-esteem and self-worth.

Attempts to pre-empt contraceptive choice by categorising contraceptive need simplistically (age, parity, social class) reflect neither the complexity of people's lives, nor the multiplicity of psychosocial factors which influence sexual relationships and reproductive choices.

For contraceptive service providers, understanding how and why people make contraceptive choices is important because minimising the likelihood of unintended pregnancy depends on maximising user satisfaction, user-effectiveness and continuation of use by providing the method that is *truly* the method of choice.

Further reading

Books

RCGP Handbook of Sexual Health in Primary Care
Eds Carter Y, Moss C and Weyman A
RCGP, 1998

Beyond Acceptability: Users' Perspectives on Contraception
Eds Ravindran Sundari T K, Berer M and Cottingham J
Reproductive Health Matters for WHO, 1997

Contraceptive choices: supporting effective use of methods
Walsh J, Lythgoe H and Peckham S
CES, **fpa**, 1996

Articles
'Consumers' understanding of contraceptive efficacy'
Godwin K
British Journal of Family Planning, 23, 1997, 45-46

'Effect of educational leaflets and questions on knowledge of contraception in women taking the combined contraceptive pill: randomised controlled trial'
Little P, Griffen S and Kelly J et al
British Medical Journal, 316, 1998, 1848-1952

'Contraceptive failure in the United States: an update'
Trussell J, Hatcher R A and Cates W, et al
Studies in Family Planning, 21, 1990, 51-54

Oral contraception

4

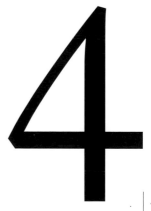

Combined oral contraceptives

General information

The combined oral contraceptive pill is one of the most effective reversible methods of contraception. *If* the pill is taken consistently, according to instructions, the chance of pregnancy occurring is practically nil. All oral contraceptives are medicinal products and they are currently (1999) supplied only on a doctor's prescription. The pill should be taken only after discussion and medical examination (blood pressure and anything that is considered relevant to the client's medical history) to exclude possible contraindications and the woman should return for regular check-ups.

Mode of action

The combined pill contains two synthetic (steroid) hormones: oestrogen and progestogen. Since its introduction in the UK in 1961, both the oestrogen and progestogen dosages have been reduced considerably to provide effective contraception while limiting unwanted side-effects. One daily pill taken in the 1960s is equivalent to seven pills taken today.

The combined pill prevents ovulation by suppressing the secretion of gonadotrophins by the hypothalamus and pituitary. In addition these pills inhibit spermatozoal transport through altered cervical mucus, prevent changes in the endometrium which are usually needed for pregnancy implantation, and interfere with normal mobility and secretion in the fallopian tubes.

Efficacy

Theoretically the pill is an extremely effective reversible method of contraception when it is taken correctly and consistently, is absorbed normally, and its metabolism is not affected by interaction with other medication. In practice, its use-effectiveness varies and pregnancy rates in general range from 0.1-7 per cent. The higher failure rates reflect lack of effective usage due to a multiplicity of factors.

Preparations available	See British National Formulary and MIMS, and Tables 3 and 4 on pages 61 and 62.

The combined pills available in the UK contain synthetic oestrogen (either ethinyloestradiol or mestranol) and a progestogen (levonorgestrel, norgestrel, ethynodiol diacetate, norethisterone, norethisterone acetate, desogestrel, gestodene or norgestimate). The progestogen levonorgestrel contains the biologically active L isomer. Other preparations contain norgestrel, a mixture of D and L isomers.

The most widely used preparations contain 30 to 40 micrograms of oestrogen or less. Occasionally preparations containing 50 micrograms of oestrogen are prescribed. No contraceptive preparations available in the UK contain more than 50 micrograms of oestrogen.

Dose

In order to minimise any possible long-term adverse effect, the recommendation from the **fpa** and the Faculty of Family Planning and Reproductive Health Care is that the pill of choice should be the one containing the lowest acceptable dose of oestrogen and progestogen which:

▶ provides effective contraception
▶ produces good menstrual cycle control
▶ is associated with fewest side-effects

Types of combined pills

Monophasic pills
Monophasic pills are the most widely used combined pills and come in packets of 21 identical tablets which are taken on 21 consecutive days. The pills are then stopped for 7 days during which some withdrawal bleeding will usually occur. After 7 pill-free days the next packet of pills is started. This routine is continued as long as contraception is required.

Phasic pills – biphasic and triphasic types
The hormone content of phasic pills varies throughout the cycle. They aim to provide a lower total dose of

hormone over each cycle. The different strengths of pill must be taken in the right order for 21 days, as marked on the packet, followed by 7 pill-free days.

Everyday (ED) pills

Everyday combined pills (ED pills) are available for those who find it easier to take pills every day without a break. Of the 28 pills, 7 are inactive, so need to be taken in the right order. There are monophasic and triphasic varieties of ED pills.

Research is continually looking into producing products that are lower in dosage, safer and easier to take. Methods with lowered oestrogen dosages, improved phasic combinations, and products with shortened pill intervals to improve usage and lower pregnancy rates, are being investigated.

Advantages
- one of the most reliable, reversible, convenient, non-intercourse related methods
- under a user's control
- often relieves painful periods (dysmenorrhoea) and may make bleeding lighter and more regular
- often relieves premenstrual symptoms
- reduces the risk of benign breast disease
- reduces the risk of fibroids and ovarian cysts
- protects against endometrial and ovarian cancer
- protects against pelvic inflammatory disease (PID)
- reduces the rate of endometriosis
- possible reduction in the risk of developing rheumatoid arthritis
- reduction in ectopic pregnancy
- decreases the risk of iron deficiency anaemia

Disadvantages
- effectiveness depends on comprehensive instruction and correct usage
- unsuitable for women with contraindications or risk factors for circulatory problems
- minor side-effects in some women when first starting the pill, such as headaches, weight gain, breakthrough bleeding

- increased incidence of some problems in some women, such as hypertension, arterial and venous disease
- not suitable for smokers over the age of 35
- problems with potential drug interactions
- effects on the breast and cervix (see page 51)
- no protection against STIs, including HIV

Absolute contra-indications

For full information see Manufacturer's Summary of Product Characteristics (SPCs).

- possible pregnancy
- abnormal vaginal or uterine bleeding of unknown cause
- cardiovascular disease, or known risk factors
- past history of thrombosis of any type (arterial or venous)
- hereditary thrombophilia (eg factor V Leiden)
- disorders of lipid metabolism
- focal or crescendo migraine or migraine requiring ergotamine treatment
- active liver disease, liver adenoma or carcinoma
- known or suspected malignancy of the breast or genital tract
- Pemphigus gestationis, deteriorating otosclerotic deafness, or cholestatic jaundice during pregnancy
- recent trophoblastic disease until elevated hCG levels are back to normal
- gall bladder disease
- psychosis or severe depression (if no other problems this can be a relative contraindication)
- two to four weeks before major or leg surgery
- ulcerative colitis (UC) or Crohn's disease with severe attacks
- porphyria
- smokers over 35 years old

The pill should only be given with special care and where appropriate with specialist advice to women who have, or have had, a first-degree relative with arterial or venous disease aged under 45, diabetes mellitus, elevated blood pressure, conditions such as epilepsy, obesity, structural heart abnormalities, renal dysfunction, or sickle cell anaemia (sickle cell trait is not a contraindication to combined pill use).

Prescribing using evidence-guided medicine

During the past four decades, much has been learnt about how the combined pill affects women. However, there are still important gaps in knowledge that relate to the pill's effect on breast and cervical cancer and effects on the vascular system. Providers need to prescribe using evidence-guided medicine, to harmonise clinical practice and avoid unnecessary interventions (screening procedures) that can be barriers for women choosing to use oral contraception.

Providers need to be aware of two initiatives aimed at improving and harmonising practice for the future:

World Health Organization (WHO)
Medical Eligibility Criteria for Contraceptive Use

Royal College of General Practitioners (RCGP)
Manchester Research Unit
Evidence-Guided Prescribing of the Pill

Work by the Reproductive Health Programme of WHO involves a new approach to classifying medical eligibility to use different contraceptive methods. This is based on the relative health risks and benefits of using a method in relation to a given illness or condition. This approach moves away from the traditional approach of identifying 'contraindications to' or 'precautions against' method use.

There are four classes of classification:

- ▶ CLASS 1 no restrictions to use – ie always usable
- ▶ CLASS 2 advantages of use outweigh theoretical or proven risk – ie unrestricted use, but selection of the type of pill is a factor
- ▶ CLASS 3 theoretical or proven risk usually outweighs advantages – ie use with caution
- ▶ CLASS 4 use not permitted at all – ie do not use

These guidelines have been produced by WHO as a reference for use with the aim that contraceptive guidelines can be harmonised.

It is hoped that this classification will help users and health professionals make improved decisions about how and why to use contraceptive methods, based on scientific rationale. This classification system has yet to be discussed and agreed by all the major family planning organisations both within the UK and outside. However, it reflects a real desire to improve overall access to safe, effective client-centred contraception.

The RCGP work resulted from the recognised need to prescribe the pill through evidence-guided medicine rather than opinion, to promote harmonisation of clinical practice, and to remove unnecessary screening interventions which lead so many women to ask:

'If the pill is so safe, why do I need all these investigations?'

The consensus from the international workshop was that only two pre-requisites were needed for the safe prescribing of the combined pill:

▶ a careful personal and family medical history with particular attention to cardiovascular risk
▶ an accurate blood pressure measurement

Further assessment is required *only* if a relevant personal or family history is disclosed, or where blood pressure is elevated.

Instructions for use of combined pills

Monophasic 21-day pills

Many preparations are available with a variety of progestogens and oestrogens in different doses. The first packet is usually started on the *first* day of bleeding (day 1 of the period) without using an additional contraceptive method. If the pill is started on any other day, an additional contraceptive method, such as the condom, *must* be used for the first 7 days after excluding any possibility of pregnancy.

Phasic combined (biphasic and triphasic) 21-day pills

The first packet is started on the *first* day of the period without the need for an additional contraceptive method. If the pill is started on any other day, an additional contraceptive method must be used for the first 7 days after excluding any possibility of pregnancy. All pills must be taken in the correct order. These pills are colour coded.

ED combined (monophasic or triphasic) 28-day pills

The first packet is started on the *first* day of the period. An additional contraceptive method must be used for the first 14 days. This is because the start day may occur with inactive not active pills. All pills must be taken every day in the correct order.

Missed pills

Ideally, oral contraceptives should be taken at a regular time each day, as their efficacy can fall if they are taken late or omitted. A combined pill is regarded as 'missed' if it is taken more than 12 hours late. If it is remembered within 12 hours, contraceptive protection is not lost. If it is taken more than 12 hours late, contraceptive protection is lost. The missed pill should be taken as soon as it is remembered. The next pill should be taken at the normal time. This may mean more than one pill is taken in one day. If more than one pill is missed, the last missed pill should be taken and the rest of the packet taken at the usual time. An extra contraceptive method must be used for 7 days. Where there are less than 7 days of pills in the pack, the pack should be finished, and a new packet should be started immediately and continued without a break. With ED pills, the 7 days of using an additional contraceptive method must include active pills to ensure contraceptive cover.

These guidelines are now the accepted standardised guidelines for missed pill advice, and have been agreed by the major oral contraceptive manufacturers and the main family planning organisations in the UK.

'Periods'

Most women who do not take the pill have menstrual cycles varying from 21 to 42 days, with 25-35 days being the average. While taking combined pills this pattern is replaced by regular withdrawal bleeds which usually follow 48-72 hours after discontinuing the last active pill. These 'periods' are usually lighter and shorter on the combined pill. Withdrawal bleeds can be postponed if bleeding will be inconvenient, and pill-taking can be adjusted. The instructions for this vary with different pills. To miss a withdrawal bleed on monophasic pills, the pills should be continued without a break (with ED pills – the inactive pills are omitted). Phasic pills are more complex, but the principle is to continue with the same or equivalent dose of progestogen to prevent a drop in hormone level. The advice here is to use the last phase of a 'spare' packet which will give, 5, 7, 10 or 14 days' postponement (depending on brand) of the withdrawal bleed. Women should be advised that in some cases breakthrough bleeding may occur, and that this is quite harmless and does not mean protection is lost. Pill cycles should not be adjusted by shortening 21-day pill-taking.

Breakthrough or irregular bleeding

Spotting or irregular bleeding is common in the first few cycles of starting the pill. If this persists beyond three months a change of pill is indicated. Women should be warned of this possibility and advised to continue pill-taking as normal, whether bleeding or not. Providing all pills have been taken as instructed, contraceptive protection is maintained.

Bleeding in a pill-taker can also be due to the following reasons, which should be considered when giving advice:

▶ default, ie missing pills
▶ very severe diarrhoea and/or vomiting
▶ drugs which interact

▶ diet (reported in a few vegetarians/vegans)
▶ disease (especially of cervix or in pregnancy,
  eg Chlamydia, cervical cancer)
▶ dose of preparation being used

Any irregular bleeding should always be investigated.

Missed 'period'

If a withdrawal bleed is missed, and the pill has been taken regularly and correctly, it is unlikely that pregnancy is the cause. If a withdrawal bleed has not occurred, the possibility of pregnancy should be considered and a pregnancy test carried out (if possible) before the next packet of pills is started. If this is not practical, the next packet should be started and a pregnancy test carried out. It is important to start the next cycle pack on time to prevent the risk of pregnancy. If two withdrawal bleeds have been missed, the next packet of pills should not be started until the possibility of pregnancy has been excluded. Pregnancy tests today allow for early diagnosis of pregnancy. Taking oral contraceptives does not alter pregnancy test results.

Smoking

It is not advisable for any woman taking oral contraceptives to smoke because of the risk of arterial disease. Women over 35 are not recommended to use combined oral contraceptive pills if they are smokers. It may be helpful to give smokers suitable literature, such as information produced by the Health Education Authority and details of the QUIT helpline (freephone 0800 002200).

Stomach upsets

Vomiting within 3 hours of taking the pill, or very severe diarrhoea, can interfere with the absorption of the pill. Women seeking simple remedies for these symptoms while on the pill should be reminded to use an additional contraceptive method (eg a condom) for any intercourse during the illness, and for 7 days of pill use after recovery (see 'Instructions for use of combined pills', page 45).

Changing pills

When changing from a higher dose preparation to a lower dose preparation, or from a combined pill to a progestogen-only pill, or vice versa, the first pill of the new packet should be taken on the next day immediately after the old packet is completed. No additional contraceptive method is necessary.

Planning a pregnancy

A woman planning a baby should stop taking the pill at the end of the packet. Ideally it is best to wait for one natural period, using another method of contraception, before trying to become pregnant. This allows the body to return to its 'pre-pill' state, allowing the pregnancy to be dated more accurately and to allow for good 'pre-pregnancy' care (see page 183). Should conception occur before this time, there is no evidence of increased birth defects, or problems with the pregnancy.

Using the pill after childbirth

Following childbirth, combined pills can be started at any time after 3 weeks postpartum (not earlier because of the increased risk of thrombosis in relation to the combined pill, and of breakthrough bleeding in relation to the progestogen-only pill). Importantly, contraception is not needed in the first 21 days after childbirth. If the combined pill is started later than 3 weeks postpartum, an extra contraceptive method should be used for the first 7 days.

Breast-feeding

Women who are breast-feeding should avoid oestrogen-containing pills as oestrogen affects lactation. Progestogen-only contraceptives are suitable, if a hormonal method is wanted.

Using the pill after a miscarriage or abortion

The combined pill can be started immediately after a first or second trimester miscarriage or abortion, as it does not interfere with recovery or increase morbidity and is effective immediately.

Operations/ surgery

Combined pills which contain oestrogen should be discontinued (and alternative contraceptive arrangements made) 2-4 weeks before major elective surgery and all surgery to the legs; they should normally be restarted on the first period occurring at least 2 weeks after mobilisation after the operation. When discontinuation is not possible, eg because of emergency surgery or if a patient admitted for an elective procedure is by oversight still on an oestrogen-containing oral contraceptive, some consideration should be given to subcutaneous heparin prophylaxis. These recommendations do not apply to minor surgery, eg tooth extractions, laparoscopy.

Using the pill after unprotected intercourse

Special doses of the pill can be used as a postcoital method within 72 hours of unprotected intercourse (see 'Postcoital contraception', page 149).

Duration of use

There is no medical evidence for routine 'breaks' in pill use. It is worth remembering that women on 21 day pills have 13 breaks, each lasting a week, every single year. Use of the pill, even for long periods of time, has not been linked to infertility. A healthy non-smoking woman with no medical contraindications can use the combined pill until the menopause.

Side-effects

Women may initially experience slight nausea, headaches, depression, breast swelling, breast tenderness, tiredness, weight increase or changes in libido. Intolerance to contact lenses may develop. Irregular (breakthrough) bleeding may occur, especially in the first month or two. These symptoms may disappear spontaneously if women are reassured and encouraged to persevere (see 'Breakthrough or irregular bleeding', page 47). Side-effects that persist should always be investigated.

Risks

The more serious side-effects, such as thrombosis or strokes, are uncommon but the risks are greater in women with the following:

▶ diabetes
▶ close relatives who have had heart attacks or strokes at an early age (under 45)

- those who are significantly overweight
- those who have elevated blood pressure
- those who smoke
- those with immobility problems (wheelchair users)

These risks increase with age and for this reason, women smokers over 35 will be discouraged from taking the combined oral contraceptive pill. Women taking the pill should in general be encouraged to stop smoking.

Combined oral contraceptives and breast and cervical cancer

Breast cancer

The literature on this is huge, complex and contradictory. Since the introduction of oral contraception, concern has centred around a possible connection with cancer. Research on breast cancer risk is complicated by problems relating to high risk groups, latency, time of exposure and changes in oral contraceptive formulation. The incidence of breast cancer in the UK is high and recognised risk factors include:

- early menarche
- late age at first birth
- family history
- diet

The 1996 publication by the Collaborative Group on Hormonal Factors in Breast Cancer re-analyses original world data from 54 studies which relates to 53,000 women with breast cancer and 100,000 controls. This represents 90 per cent of the world's epidemiological data on this subject. The clear conclusion of this study is that there is a small increase in risk of having breast cancer diagnosed during pill use and for 10 years thereafter. There is no increased risk 10 or more years after stopping use. In absolute terms, the excess risk is 0.5 cancers per 10,000 women who used the pill at 16-19 and this increases with age. See Table 2, *Cumulative risk of breast cancer by recency of use.*

Table 2 Cumulative risk of breast cancer by recency of use
numbers per 10,000

	to age 20	to age 25	to age 30	to age 35	to age 40	to age 45
Breast cancer diagnosed by	age 30	age 35	age 40	age 45	age 50	age 55
Never-users	4	16	44	100	160	230
Pill-users who stopped 10 years earlier	4.5	17.5	49	110	180	260
Excess number of breast cancer per 10,000 women	0.5	1.5	5	10	20	30

The cancers diagnosed in women who use or have used the pill are clinically less advanced than those who have never used the pill, and are less likely to have spread beyond the breast. The re-analysis shows that risks are *not* associated with duration of use, the dose or type of hormone in the pill or family history. The authors of the study comment that it is not possible to infer from the data whether the risk is due to an earlier diagnosis of breast cancer in ever users, the biological effects of hormonal contraceptives, or a combination of reasons.

It is always important that pill users should be advised of all risks and benefits and any uncertainties. All information and advice should be explicitly supported by the best available evidence and should be discussed in relation to each individual.

Cervical cancer
With regard to cervical cancer, sexual behaviour (age at first intercourse, number of sexual partners), multiple pregnancies, cigarette smoking, sexually transmitted infections (STIs) and socio-economic status are important determinants of cancer of the cervix. The literature looking at oral contraceptive use and squamous cervical cancer is not clear. Recent studies suggest the pill may be a weak co-factor in causing cervical cancer. However, the many confounding factors make this unclear. The prime carcinogen is likely to be sexually transmitted,

probably a virus or combination of viruses. Pill users should be screened following the national cervical cytology guidelines. In the presence of any abnormality, the combined pill may be used with monitoring. Adenocarcinoma and adenosquamous carcinoma are rare cancers of the cervix. Studies are continuing to look into the effects that oral contraceptives may have on these cancers.

Combined oral contraceptives and cardiovascular disease

Despite known clear and substantial benefits of the pill, concern has remained about its short-term and long-term effects on the increased risk of venous thromboembolism, myocardial infarction and stroke (ischaemic and haemorrhagic). As a result of this concern, oral contraceptives continue to be refined with respect to dosage and constituent.

Combined oral contraceptives and thrombo-embolism

For many years it has been known that women who use combined oral contraceptives have an increased risk of venous thromboembolism. The increased risk is small, is present only while women use the pill and is unrelated to duration of use. Studies published in 1995/96 showed that users of pills containing the progestogens gestodene and desogestrel have twice the risk of venous thrombosis compared with users of pills containing levonorgestrel, norethisterone or ethynodiol. (Risk of venous thrombosis in a never-user of the pill is five per 100,000 women, in a pregnant woman it is 60 per 100,000 women, in combined pills containing gestodene and desogestrel it is 30 per 100,000 women, and in pills containing levonorgestrel/norethisterone it is 15 per 100,000 women.) There are few data available concerning the risk of venous thrombosis with pills containing norgestimate.

Only one to two per cent of these thromboses will be fatal. The excess risk is considered to be small and needs to be weighed up against other prescribing factors. The original hypothesis with the introduction of the newer progestogens was that they would offer beneficial effects on the risk of myocardial infarction and other arterial system damage for pill users. Data from clinical use are not yet available to confirm this hypothesis.

The Committee on Safety of Medicines recommends that oral contraceptives containing the progestogens gestodene or desogestrel should only be used when there are specific reasons to do so in an individual case, and that all women taking these preparations should understand that there is an associated increased risk of venous thromboembolism, compared to using other combined oral contraceptives.

Combined oral contraceptives and stroke

The increased risk of cerebrovascular accidents (strokes) in combined pill users has been known since the early 1960s. Consistent research findings since that time have suggested a true association between combined pill use and stroke.

WHO data published in 1996 looking at more than 8,000 women using the combined pill, confirm previous research and show that the absolute risk of stroke is small. The incidence of ischaemic stroke is low and any risk attributable to use of the pill is small. Haemorrhagic stroke is slightly increased in combined pill users. Risk of all types of stroke is increased by factors such as oestrogen dose, raised blood pressure, age (over 35) and smoking.

This research confirms the need for good blood pressure monitoring in pill users before and during use, and advice to stop smoking.

Other symptoms

Although women should be made aware of the risks of the pill, it must be emphasised that the number of women who actually encounter problems is extremely small, and for most women the benefits of the pill outweigh the possible disadvantages.

For a fuller review of side-effects see 'Further reading' on pages 69-72.

Women should be investigated immediately if they develop any of the following:

- ► painful swelling of a leg(s)
- ► pain in the chest or abdomen
- ► breathlessness or cough with blood-stained phlegm
- ► a bad fainting attack or collapse
- ► unusual headache or disturbance of speech or eyesight
- ► numbness or weakness of a limb
- ► jaundice (yellow skin or yellow eyes)
- ► severe and generalised skin rash

Symptoms such as lumps in the breast, discharge from a nipple, or bleeding after sexual intercourse should be investigated promptly.

Combined oral contraceptives and drugs

Pill efficacy may in some instances be reduced by concurrent medication, due to mechanisms that reduce the bioavailability of oestrogen or progestogen in the body. In addition, the pill may sometimes modify the action of a particular drug being taken. This section will only address drugs and reduced efficacy of the pill.

Bioavailability is the extent to which a drug reaches or has access to its site of action from the bloodstream. The bioavailability of hormonal contraceptives is affected by their metabolism in the liver. Oestrogen and progestogens are metabolised in the liver into active metabolites which are excreted. The bioavailability of combined oral contraceptives is also influenced by reabsorption of ethinyloestradiol from the bowel. This process is called enterohepatic recycling. Any mechanism that affects this will alter contraceptive efficacy.

Certain drugs are known to reduce the efficacy of the pill in some women. Pregnancies have occurred as a result of interactions between the pill and antibacterials as well as anticonvulsant drugs. Although the evidence for reduced efficacy of the pill with broad spectrum antibiotics is based on small numbers, it is prudent to recommend additional contraceptive cover for women taking certain antibiotics and the pill. This is particularly important when liver enzyme inducers, especially rifampicin, griseofulvin, and some anticonvulsants are taken as these significantly reduce blood concentrations of both oestrogen and progestogen.

The main drugs which may reduce the efficacy of the combined pill

CNS active-drugs: anticonvulsant drugs, barbiturates, CNS stimulant

Many common anticonvulsants induce hepatic drug metabolising enzymes thereby lowering levels of both oestrogen and progestogen. Topiramate, a new anti-convulsant drug, is an enzyme inducing drug. Other newer drugs such as vigabatrin, lamotrigine and clobazam do not have this property and neither do older drugs such as sodium valproate and clonazepam.

A number of pregnancies have been reported in women receiving the combined pill and:

▶ Phenobarbitone   ▶ Primidone
▶ Hydantoins (phenytoin)   ▶ Carbamazepine

Barbiturates, and to a lesser extent, hydantoins and primidone are microsomal enzyme inducers in humans, and may increase the rate of metabolism of contraceptive steroids.

Advice
A higher dose of ethinyloestradiol containing 50mcg or more is advisable if alternative methods of contraception are inappropriate for women with epilepsy. It is also suggested that the recommendation of 'tricycling' using monophasic pills is useful for some women. This involves taking three or four packets in a row followed by a short pill-free interval of 4 days. This reduces the number of pill-free episodes. Caution is advised when enzyme inducers are withdrawn, since it takes some time for the liver's level of excretory function to revert to normal. Advice needs to be taken on how long extra contraceptive

cover is required after drug therapy. Medical opinion suggests 4 weeks' cover is required depending on the type of enzyme inducer used.

Antituberculous drugs

Rifampicin and rifabutin are potent enzyme inducing drugs. Most women using oral contraceptives concurrently with these have poor cycle control (ie irregular bleeding). Some pregnancies have been reported. Therefore it is normal practice always to advise an alternative method of contraception when women are taking these over a prolonged time. Short-term use of rifampicin/rifabutin (ie a short course to clear meningococci from the nose or for TB prophylaxis) also requires additional contraceptive precautions over this time *and* for 4 weeks after.

Antifungals/antibacterials

A small number of pregnancies have occurred in women taking combined oral contraceptives and

antifungals:
► Griseofulvin (see information on enzyme inducers).

antibacterials
including:
► Ampicillin   ► Amoxycillin   ► Augmentin
► Tetracyclines   ► Cephalosporins
► Rifampicin/rifabutin (see antituberculous drugs and information on enzyme inducers)

Doxycycline (a tetracycline) is now being recommended and prescribed as an anti-malarial for people travelling to areas where the usual anti-malarials are no longer effective. Recognised anti-malarial drugs do not interfere with oral contraceptives, but doxycycline may, so any general question on anti-malarials should check whether doxycycline has been prescribed.

Advice

Broad spectrum antibiotics interact only with oestrogen (so the progestogen-only pill is unaffected). Certain antibiotics appear to alter the colonic flora and reduce their capacity to hydrolyse oestrogen conjugates in the bowel back into active oestrogen, so reducing plasma levels. Despite anecdotal evidence, there is no established proof that non-enzyme inducing antibiotics do decrease the efficacy of the combined pill. Based on biochemical and clinical data it is almost certain that erythromycin, cotrimoxazole and sulphonamides do not interact with the combined pill. However, as uncertainty remains with other antibiotics (particularly penicillins and tetracyclines), use of an additional contraceptive method is recommended where these drugs are prescribed.

The recommended clinical advice is that women on the pill should use additional contraceptive cover during all short courses (2 weeks or less) of these antibiotics, and for 7 days after the last antibiotic tablet. If the 7 days run beyond the end of a packet then a new packet should be started immediately and continued without a break. With ED pills the inactive pills should be missed out (see 'Instructions for use of combined pills', page 45). If such an antibiotic is continued for 2 weeks or more, the flora develop resistance and oestrogen levels rise back to normal. Thus women who have taken long-term antibiotics for at least 3 weeks, eg for acne, need not take extra contraceptive precautions. Combined pill users who start a long-term course of antibiotics (for example tetracyclines) should use an additional contraceptive method for 3 weeks. Women who are already on long-term antibiotics (ie have used them for 3 weeks or more) prior to starting COCs do not need additional contraception.

Effects of combined oral contraceptives on other drugs

The combined pill slightly lowers the clearance of diazepam, prednisolone and probably other drugs. This may increase the risk of side-effects, but is considered to be clinically insignificant. It also impairs the metabolism of warfarin and alters clotting factors. As the interaction is unpredictable, this combination of drugs should be avoided.

Recreational drugs

Breakthrough bleeding has been reported while using the combined pill and recreational drugs. There is, however, no pharmacological basis for such an interaction. The irregular bleeding is often due to poor pill-taking.

Vitamins

There is no reduction in the efficiency of the combined pill if a woman is also taking vitamin supplements.

For a full review of drugs and oral contraceptives see British National Formulary, and 'Further reading' on pages 69-72.

Anti-androgen pills

Dianette

Dianette is an anti-androgen/oestrogen combination for the oral treatment of acne, seborrhoea and mild hirsutism in women and is also a reliable contraceptive. Dianette contains 2mg cyproterone acetate and 35mcg ethinyl-oestradiol in packs of 21 tablets. It is not primarily prescribed for contraception and not often available in community family planning clinics.

General follow-up

Women should be seen as instructed, this is usually every 6 months. Where a prescription is written for 13 months, a woman should be seen where possible after at least 6 months. This gives an opportunity to check that the method is still appropriate and is being used correctly.

Follow-up assessment should enquire about any questions and concerns the woman might have, and any new risk factors which might have developed, such as headaches or migraine.

Routine physical checks should be kept to a *minimum.* Blood pressure should be monitored, comparing it to a baseline recording taken when the pill was first prescribed.

Available data do not support regular screening that includes periodic pelvic examination (perineum, vagina, cervix, anus) and cervical cytology as procedures *necessary for combined oral contraceptive use.* They are, however, recommended for women who are sexually active and as such any procedure carried out should be explained as to *what* it is and *why* it is being offered.

Women should always be encouraged to ask their family doctor or clinic if they have any worries or concerns about any aspect of pill-taking.

Table 3 Monophasic combined oral contraceptives

Pill type & preparation	Manufacturer	Oestrogen (mcg)	Progestogen (mg)	
Combined – monophasic				
Ethinyloestradiol / norethisterone type				
Loestrin 20	Parke-Davis	20	1	norethisterone acetate
Loestrin 30	Parke-Davis	30	1.5	norethisterone acetate
Brevinor	Searle	35	0.5	norethisterone
Ovysmen	Janssen-Cilag	35	0.5	norethisterone
Norimin	Searle	35	1	norethisterone
Ethinyloestradiol / levonorgestrel				
Microgynon 30 (also ED)	Schering HC	30	0.15	
Ovranette	Wyeth	30	0.15	
Eugynon 30	Schering HC	30	0.25	
Ovran 30	Wyeth	30	0.25	
Ovran	Wyeth	50	0.25	
Ethinyloestradiol / desogestrel				
Mercilon	Organon	20	0.15	
Marvelon	Organon	30	0.15	
Ethinyloestradiol / gestodene				
Femodene (also ED)	Schering HC	30	0.075	
Minulet	Wyeth	30	0.075	
Ethinyloestradiol / norgestimate				
Cilest	Janssen-Cilag	35	0.25	
Mestranol / norethisterone				
Norinyl-1	Searle	50	1	
Ortho-Novin 1/50	Janssen-Cilag	50	1	

Reproduced with permission of MIMS 1998

Table 4 Phasic combined oral contraceptives

Pill type & preparation	Manufacturer	Oestrogen (mcg)	Progestogen (mg)	
Biphasic & Triphasic				
Ethinyloestradiol / norethisterone				
BiNovum	Janssen-Cilag	35	0.5	(7 tabs)
		35	1	(14 tabs)
Synphase	Searle	35	0.5	(7 tabs)
		35	1	(9 tabs)
		35	0.5	(5 tabs)
TriNovum	Janssen-Cilag	35	0.5	(7 tabs)
		35	0.75	(7 tabs)
		35	1	(7 tabs)
Ethinyloestradiol / levonorgestrel				
Logynon (also ED)	Schering HC	30	0.05	(6 tabs)
		40	0.075	(5 tabs)
		30	0.125	(10 tabs)
Trinordiol	Wyeth	30	0.05	(6 tabs)
		40	0.075	(5 tabs)
		30	0.125	(10 tabs)
Ethinyloestradiol / gestodene				
Tri-Minulet	Wyeth	30	0.05	(6 tabs)
		40	0.07	(5 tabs)
		30	0.1	(10 tabs)
Triadene	Schering HC	30	0.05	(6 tabs)
		40	0.07	(5 tabs)
		30	0.1	(10 tabs)

Reproduced with permission of MIMS 1998

Progestogen-only pills

General information

Progestogen-only pills (POPs) contain no oestrogen. They contain progestogen only. They are a useful alternative for women wishing to use oral contraception who choose not to use oestrogen or where oestrogens are contraindicated, such as women over 35 years who smoke and breast-feeding mothers.

Mode of action

The progestogen-only pill does not always prevent ovulation. (It prevents ovulation in 15-40 per cent of cycles.) Progestogen acts on the cervical mucus, endometrium and fallopian tubes, causing changes that make it difficult for sperm to enter the womb, and rendering the lining of the womb unreceptive to the egg if fertilised.

Efficacy

The progestogen-only pill, contrary to professional and public opinion, is a very effective method of contraception when taken correctly and consistently. In practice, its use-effectiveness varies and pregnancy rates range from 1-10 per cent. The higher failure rates reflect lack of effective usage due to a multiplicity of factors. Some research suggests that the efficacy rate of progestogen-only methods is reduced in some women weighing over 70kg (11 stones). The clinical significance of this is being further investigated.

Preparations available

See British National Formulary (section 7.3.2) and MIMS, and Table 5.

Progestogen-only pills contain low doses of the following progestogens: norethisterone, ethynodiol diacetate (converts to norethisterone) or levonorgestrel.

Advantages

▶ easy and convenient to use
▶ non-intercourse related method
▶ suitable for older women who smoke and those who are breast-feeding

▶ suitable for women who cannot use oestrogen-containing oral contraceptives

▶ minimal alteration in carbohydrate and lipid metabolism

▶ no evidence of increased risk of cardiovascular disease, thromboembolism or hypertension

▶ may relieve premenstrual tension and dysmenorrhoea

Disadvantages

▶ not as effective as combined pills

▶ must be taken at a regular time to achieve optimum effectiveness

▶ disruption of menstrual pattern including increased spotting, breakthrough bleeding or amenorrhoea

▶ possible increase in ectopic pregnancy in the event of POP failure

▶ a small number of women will develop functional ovarian cysts

Contra-indications

For full information see Manufacturer's Summary of Product Characteristics (SPCs).

▶ possible pregnancy

▶ abnormal vaginal or uterine bleeding of unknown cause

▶ previous ectopic pregnancy

▶ recent trophoblastic disease until elevated hCG levels are back to normal

▶ any known malignant disease of the breast

▶ active liver disease, liver adenoma or carcinoma

▶ recurrent cholestatic jaundice

▶ history of jaundice in pregnancy (relative contraindication)

▶ past severe arterial disease or severely abnormal lipid profile

▶ any serious side-effects from use of combined oral contraceptives which were not attributed to oestrogen

▶ past hospitalisation for functional ovarian cysts

▶ unacceptability of irregular menstrual bleeding

Instructions for use of progestogen-only pills

The first packet is started on the first day (day 1) of the period without the need for additional contraceptive cover and then taken daily, without a break, even through the period.

It is important that the pill is taken at the same time each day as the efficiency falls markedly if tablets are taken late or omitted. A progestogen-only pill is regarded as 'missed' if taken only 3 hours late. In such cases, the missed pill should be taken immediately and normal pill-taking resumed when the next pill is due. Additional contraceptive precautions should be taken for 7 days. Before 1993, the guideline for additional contraceptive precautions was 48 hours. This change allows for standardisation of guidelines between combined oral contraceptives and progestogen-only contraception. It should be noted that although this 7-day advice increases consensus and consistency it does not add any important additional efficacy to the previous 48-hour recommendation. The main family planning organisations and the contraceptive manufacturers continue to work together to produce common agreed guidelines on all methods of contraception based on current research and informed opinion, in order that users and potential users receive harmonised information.

Periods

Changes in the menstrual cycle are quite common in progestogen-only pill users. Menstrual irregularity is the main problem with progestogen-only methods. This sometimes settles down after a few cycles. Spotting and breakthrough bleeding also occur in some women. For some, periods stop completely. Providing pregnancy is excluded this problem is not harmful and implies that ovulation is being inhibited. If such changes are not acceptable, a change of pill or method is usually indicated.

Smoking

Although it is not advisable for any woman to smoke, smoking is not a contraindication to progestogen-only pills.

Stomach upsets

Vomiting within 3 hours of taking the pill, or very severe diarrhoea can interfere with absorption of the pill. An additional contraceptive method should be used over the time of illness and for 7 days after recovery. (See 'Instructions for use of progestogen-only pills', page 64.)

Changing pills

When changing from one progestogen-only pill to another, or from a combined oral contraceptive pill to a progestogen-only pill, or vice versa, the first pill of the new pack should be started on the next day immediately after the old pack is complete. No additional contraceptive method is necessary.

Planning a pregnancy

A woman planning a baby should stop taking the pill at the end of the pack. Ideally it is best to wait for one natural period using another method of contraception, before trying to become pregnant. This allows the body to return to its 'pre-pill' state, allowing the pregnancy to be dated more accurately and to allow for good 'pre-pregnancy' care (see page 183). Should conception occur before this time, there is no evidence of increased birth defects, or problems with the pregnancy.

Using the pill after childbirth and while breast-feeding

Progestogen-only pills can be taken from day 21 after childbirth. Use before day 21 causes an increase in irregular bleeding and, importantly, contraception is not needed in the first 21 days after childbirth. This pill is not contraindicated for breast-feeding mothers. Most studies have failed to demonstrate any alteration in the quality or quantity of milk. Although a small amount of progestogen may be ingested by the baby, extensive research shows no evidence of any deleterious effects.

Using the pill after a miscarriage or abortion

The progestogen-only pill can be started immediately after a first or second trimester miscarriage or abortion, as it does not interfere with recovery or increase morbidity and is effective immediately.

Operations/ surgery

Progestogen-only preparations need not be discontinued if surgery is needed.

Side-effects

The main side-effect of progestogen-only pills is menstrual irregularity (see 'Periods', page 65). Other effects include weight gain, breast tenderness, decreased libido, acne and headaches in some women. These symptoms usually settle down after the first few cycles.

Risks

The proportion of ectopic pregnancies (ie where the pregnancy develops outside the uterus, usually in a fallopian tube), is increased in progestogen-only pill users, but the incidence is low and much less than would be expected in women not using contraception. Any ectopic pregnancy that does occur is due to the fact that progestogen-only pills are more effective at limiting intrauterine rather than extrauterine pregnancies. The possibility of ectopic pregnancy must always be considered in any woman who develops sudden lower abdominal pain, with a light, scanty or missed period. Women using progestogen-only methods also have increased risk of functional ovarian cysts. These may cause pain, or may not cause any problems. They are not dangerous and do not require surgery. These cysts usually disappear without treatment, but may require monitoring.

Progestogen-only pills and breast cancer

The 1996 Collaborative Group on Hormonal Factors in Breast Cancer Study (see 'Combined oral contraceptives and breast and cervical cancer', page 51) found that risk factors for progestogen-only pill users were similar for those using the combined pill with some evidence of an increased risk for use in the previous five years. There was no evidence of an increase in risk 10 years or more after stopping the progestogen-only pill. However as the number of POP users was very small in this study (0.8 per cent of the study population), these data should be interpreted with care.

Drug interactions with progestogen-only pills

See 'Combined oral contraceptives and drugs', page 55. However, it is important to note that there is no interaction between antibiotics and progestogen-only pills.

67

Table 5 Progestogen-only oral contraceptives

Pill type & preparation	Manufacturer	Progestogen (mg)	
Norethisterone type			
Micronor	Janssen-Cilag	0.35	norethisterone
Noriday	Searle	0.35	norethisterone
Femulen	Searle	0.5	ethynodiol diacetate*
Levonorgestrel			
Microval	Wyeth	0.03	
Norgeston	Schering HC	0.03	
Neogest	Schering HC	0.075	norgestrel

*Converted (> 90%) to norethisterone as the active metabolite

Reproduced with permission of MIMS 1998

Further reading

Books

The pill
Guillebaud J
5th edn, Oxford University Press, 1997

Summary of drug interactions with oral contraception
Guerts T B P, Goorissen E M and Sitsen J M A
Parthenon Publishing Group, 1993

Contraception – your questions answered
Guillebaud J
2nd edn, Churchill Livingstone, 1993 (revised 1994),
new edition due mid 1999
Chapter 4: Oral contraception – the combined oral
contraceptive (COC)
Chapter 5: Oestrogen-free hormonal contraception

Pharmacology of the contraceptive steroids
Goldzieher J W (chief editor)
Raven Press, New York, 1994

*Handbook of family planning and reproductive
health care*
Loudon N, Glasier A and Gebbie A (eds)
3rd edn, Churchill Livingstone, 1995
Chapter 3: Combined hormonal contraception,
Guillebaud J
Chapter 4: Progestogen-only contraception, Fraser I

Evidence-guided prescribing of the pill
RCGP Manchester Research Unit
Hannaford P C and Webb A M C (eds)
Parthenon Publishing Group, 1996

*Improving access to quality care in family planning:
medical eligibility criteria for contraceptive use*
WHO, Geneva, 1996

Articles

'Do combined oral contraceptive users know how to take their pill correctly?'
Brook S J and Smith C
British Journal of Family Planning, 17, 1991, 18-20

'Venous thromboembolic disease and combined oral contraceptives: results of an international multicentre case-control study'
WHO Collaborative Study of Cardiovascular Disease and Steroid Hormone Contraception
Poulter N R, Chang C L and Farley T M M, et al
The Lancet, 346, 1995, 1575-82

'Effect of different progestogens in low oestrogen oral contraceptives on venous thromboembolic disease'
WHO Collaborative Study of Cardiovascular Disease and Steroid Hormone Contraception
Farley T M M, Meirik O and Chang C L, et al
The Lancet, 346, 1995, 1582-88

'Enhancement of factor V Leiden mutation of risk of deep-vein thrombosis associated with oral contraceptives containing a third-generation progestogen'
Bloemenkamp K W M, Rosendaal F R and Helmerhorst F M, et al
The Lancet, 346, 1995, 1589-93

'Third generation oral contraceptives and risk of venous thromboembolic disorders: an international case-control study'
Transnational Research Group on Oral Contraceptives and the Health of Young Women
Spitzer W D, Lewis M A, and Heineman L A J, et al
British Medical Journal, 312, 1996, 83-88

'The increased risk of venous thromboembolism and the use of third generation progestogens: role of bias in observational research'
Lewis M A, Lothar A J and Heinemann K D, et al
Contraception, 54, 1996, 5-13

'Breast cancer and hormonal contraceptives: collaborative reanalysis of individual data of 53,294 women with breast cancer and 100,239 women without breast cancer from 54 epidemiological studies'
Collaborative Group on Hormonal Factors in Breast Cancer
The Lancet, 347, 1996, 1713-27

'Ischaemic stroke and combined oral contraceptives: results of an international, multicentre, case-control study'
WHO Collaborative Study on Cardiovascular Disease and Steroid Hormone Contraception
The Lancet, 348, 1996, 498-505

'Haemorrhagic stroke, overall stroke risk and combined oral contraceptives: results of an international, multi-centre, case-control study'
WHO Collaborative Study on Cardiovascular Disease and Steroid Hormone Contraception
The Lancet, 348, 1996, 505-10

'The effects on mortality of the use of combined oral contraceptives'
Oldfield K, Milne R and Vessey M
British Journal of Family Planning, 24, 1998, 2-6

'Combined oral contraceptives, migraine and ischaemic stroke: Recommendations for Clinical Practice'
MacGregor A E and Guillebaud J in conjunction with The Faculty of Family Planning and Reproductive Health Care of the RCOG and the **fpa**
British Journal of Family Planning, 24, 1998, 53-60

'The risk of serious illness among oral contraceptive users: evidence from the RCGP's oral contraceptive study'
Hannaford P C and Kay CR
British Journal of General Practice, 48, 1998, 1657-62

'Risk of myocordial infarction, angina and stroke in users of oral contraceptives: an updated analysis of a cohort study'
Mant J, Painter R, Vessey M
British Journal of Obstetrics and Gynaecology, 105, 1998, 890-96

'Mortality associated with oral contraceptive use: 25 years follow up of cohort of 46,000 women from the Royal College of General Practitioners' Oral Contraception Study'
Beral V, Hermon C, Kay C et al
British Medical Journal, 318, 1999, 96-100

International consensus statement

'Evidence-guided prescribing of combined oral contraceptives: consensus statement'
Hannaford P C and Webb A M C
Contraception, 54, 1996, 125-29

Injectable contraception

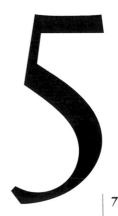

General information

There are two injectable contraceptive methods in the UK: Depo-Provera (medroxyprogesterone acetate) and Noristerat (norethisterone oenanthate).

Mode of action

Injectables work in a similar way to the progestogen-only pill, but in addition always inhibit ovulation. Both injectable preparations are given as deep intramuscular injection within the first 5 days of menstruation and are effective immediately. If given after this time an additional method of contraception should be used for 7 days. Depo-Provera is given every 12 weeks and Noristerat is repeated once after 8 weeks.

Effectiveness

Both Depo-Provera and Noristerat are highly effective methods of contraception. A main advantage is no 'user' failures. The efficacy rate is 99 to almost 100 per cent (0.1-0.6 per cent failure).

Table 6 Injectable contraceptive products

Product & manufacturer	Chemical constituents	Dosage	Presentation
Depo-Provera (150 mg/ml) Pharmacia & Upjohn	medroxyprogesterone acetate	A single injection of 150mg i.m. every 12 weeks	A sterile aqueous suspension of medroxyprogesterone acetate: 150 mg/ml suspended in pre-filled syringe -1 ml
Noristerat Schering HC	norethisterone oenanthate	A single injection of 200mg i.m. repeated once after 8 weeks	200 mg/ml in a vehicle of benzyl benzoate and castor oil in 1 ml ampoules

Licensing in the UK

Depo-Provera

Depot-medroxyprogesterone acetate (DMPA) was licensed for short-term use until 1984. A long-term licence for Depo-Provera was granted in the same year for use by women for whom other contraceptives are contraindicated, have caused unacceptable side-effects or are otherwise unsatisfactory.

This method is now available in over 90 countries, including the USA, and today is available as a first choice method, not just for women who cannot use other methods.

Noristerat

Noristerat is presently licensed only for short-term use (two injections only) for women whose partners have undergone vasectomy until the vasectomy is effective, and for women immunised against rubella, to prevent pregnancy during the active period of the virus.

Advantages

► very effective method of family planning
► one injection lasts for 8-12 weeks (depending on type)
► non-intercourse related method
► helpful for women with premenstrual symptoms and painful periods
► safe; no deaths associated with this method
► minimal metabolic effects
► no association with cardiovascular disease
► can be used by breast-feeding mothers
► most of the non-contraceptive benefits of combined oral contraceptives, including protection against PID and reduction in the risk of endometrial cancer

Disadvantages

► menstrual disturbances – bleeding may be frequent, irregular or absent
► weight gain (mainly associated with Depo-Provera)
► a long delay in the return of fertility (up to a year or more with Depo-Provera), although the method is fully reversible
► depression in some women
► cannot be withdrawn once administered

Contra-indications

For full information see Manufacturer's Summary of Product Characteristics (SPCs).

Injectable methods should not be given to women with:

► possible pregnancy
► cancer of the breast or undiagnosed breast lump
► all genital cancers (except as treatment for endometrial cancer)
► undiagnosed vaginal or uterine bleeding

▶ past severe arterial disease or current very high risk or severely abnormal lipid profile

▶ recent trophoblastic disease until elevated hCG levels are back to normal

▶ active liver disease, liver adenoma or carcinoma

▶ serious side-effects on combined oral contraceptives, not clearly oestrogen attributable

▶ those who cannot accept menstrual irregularity

▶ progestogen-sensitive migraine

▶ those wishing to conceive immediately after use of the injectable method

Periods

Most women using progestogen-only preparations experience some menstrual disturbance, which is not harmful. Injectables can cause irregular periods, spotting between periods or complete absence of periods (particularly after two or more injections). Menstrual irregularity is the main reason for discontinuation of this method. Women should be fully counselled about this when choosing injectable preparations.

Side-effects

The main reported side-effects include menstrual disturbances (see 'Periods' above), weight gain, headaches, some fluid retention, changes in mood, libido and depression in some women. Rare cases of thrombosis have been reported, but causality has not been established.

Injectable contraception and breast and cervical cancer

Breast cancer

The 1996 Collaborative Group on Hormonal Factors in Breast Cancer Study (see 'Combined oral contraceptives and breast and cervical cancer', page 51) found that risk factors for injectable contraceptive method users were similar to those using oral contraceptives, with some evidence of an increased risk for use in the previous five years. There was no evidence of an increase in risk 10 years or more after stopping injectable methods. However, as the number of injectable contraceptive method users was small (1.5 per cent of the study population), these data should be interpreted with care.

Cervical cancer

Research shows no increased risk of invasive cervical cancer among women who have used DMPA, even those who have used it for long periods of time. However, causal factors relating to cancer of the cervix are difficult to determine because of the multiplicity of factors. Hormonal contraception, including DMPA, may have a promoting role. Further study is ongoing to clarify the situation.

There are no data from human studies on Noristerat and cancer.

Bone mineral density changes

Data in 1994, from a very small cross-sectional study, suggested that use of Depo-Provera may be a risk factor for osteoporosis. New research in 1998 now suggests that long-term use of Depo-Provera shows no clinically important adverse effects on bone density. There is no evidence to recommend add-back oestrogen in Depo-Provera users in relation to osteoporosis. More research is required about possible prolonged hypo-oestrogenism in long-term Depo-Provera users.

Planning a pregnancy

Many women experience a delay of return to fertility (more so with Depo-Provera) of up to a year or more. Once cycles have returned regularly after stopping injections, there is no evidence of Depo-Provera causing infertility. It should be noted that there is always a varying interval between women deciding to become pregnant and actual conception.

After childbirth and while breast-feeding

Because of the risk of heavy or prolonged bleeding in some women, it is recommended that injectable methods in general should not be used until 5 to 6 weeks after childbirth. Injectable methods may safely be used while breast-feeding. Research on Depo-Provera has shown no deleterious effects on babies or infant growth or morbidity.

After a miscarriage or abortion

Injectable progestogens can be started immediately after first or second trimester miscarriage or abortion, as they do not affect recovery or increase morbidity and are effective immediately.

Drug interactions

There are little data on injectable methods and it is not known if injectable methods are affected by other medication in the same way as oral contraceptives. However, progestogens are known to be affected by enzyme inducing drugs (see 'Combined oral contraceptives and drugs', page 55). Women taking enzyme inducing drugs should have their injection frequency increased from 12 to 10 weeks for Depo-Provera and from 8 to 6 weeks for Noristerat.

Monthly injectables and future methods

Research into improving injectable methods has been going on since the 1960s. Monthly injectables are available in some parts of the world.

► Cyclofem/Cycloprovera contains 25mg of medroxyprogesterone acetate and 5mg of oestradiol cypionate.

► Mesigyna contains 50mg of norethisterone oenanthate and 5mg of oestradiol valerate.

The World Health Organization is currently researching a number of different preparations.

Further reading

Books

Contraception – your questions answered
Guillebaud J
2nd edn, Churchill Livingstone, 1993 (revised 1994)
Chapter 5: Oestrogen-free hormonal contraception

Handbook of family planning and reproductive health care
Loudon N, Glasier A and Gebbie A (eds)
3rd edn, Churchill Livingstone, 1995
Chapter 4: Progestogen-only contraception, Fraser I

Articles

'Recovery of bone density in women who stop using medroxyprogesterone acetate'
Cundy T, Cornish J and Evans M C, et al
British Medical Journal, 308, 1994, 247-48

'Bone density in long-term users of depot medroxy-progesterone acetate'
Gbolade B, Ellis S and Murby B, et al
British Journal of Obstetrics and Gynaecology, 105, 1998, 790-94

Contraceptive implants

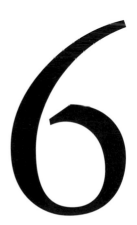

**General
information**

Contraceptive implants offer an alternative way of delivering hormones that are long-acting, low-dose and reversible methods of contraception. A wide range of materials and approaches has been used in the development of different hormonal delivery systems. Levonorgestrel is the most widely used hormone to date, but the newer progestogens may also prove valuable in the future.

Norplant, the first contraceptive implant, became available in the UK in 1993. This implant is widely used in other countries and the number of users worldwide exceeds two million women. Norplant is available in the same way as other contraceptive methods. Specialised training is essential for the success of this method. Training is organised by the FFPRHC. The Letter of Competence in Subdermal Contraceptive Implants includes completion of removal training. Training is available for doctors and nurses.

Objective information about Norplant's risks and benefits is reassuring; the introduction of this new method was welcomed and considered successful. However, considerable adverse publicity based on anecdotal cases of difficulties with Norplant in the US and UK have led to legal concerns, considerable publicity and wariness by the public and professionals.

Norplant consists of six thin flexible rods made of soft silastic. Each implant measures 34mm in length and 2.44mm in diameter. Each contains 38mg of levonorgestrel.

Using local anaesthesia, Norplant is inserted subdermally through a small incision (3-5mm) using a purpose-designed trocar. The rods are positioned carefully in a fan shape in the inner aspect of the non-dominant arm, approximately 6-8cm above the fold of the elbow. Strict asepsis must be observed. Different insertion techniques are likely to be developed for newer systems.

Once the implant is in place it is effective for 5 years. The implant can be removed at any time during this period. Women should be reassured that the implants are not breakable.

Implanon is being introduced into the UK in 1999. Implanon is a single ethylene vinylacetate rod measuring 40mm by 2mm. It contains 68mg etonogestrel. The rod is preloaded into a sterile, single-use applicator. It is inserted subdermally on the inner aspect of the upper arm. Once in place it is effective for 3 years. Implanon must be inserted and removed only by trained professionals.

Mode of action   Contraceptive implants work by preventing ovulation in about 50 per cent of menstrual cycles by thickening the cervical mucus, preventing sperm penetration and by suppression of the endometrium.

Efficacy   Contraceptive implants are highly effective. Norplant is over 99 per cent effective in the first year of use, and about 98 per cent effective over 5 years. Early trial data show no pregnancies with Implanon (December 1998).

Time of insertion   Implants can be inserted during the first five days of the menstrual cycle. No additional contraceptive methods are needed. If inserted after this time, an additional contraceptive method is required for the first 7 days.

Advantages
▶ long-lasting
▶ very effective
▶ reversible and no effect on future fertility
▶ non-intercourse related
▶ free from oestrogen side-effects
▶ requires little medical attention other than at insertion and removal

Disadvantages
▶ requires a minor operative procedure
▶ irregular menstrual bleeding may occur
▶ possible risk of ectopic pregnancy (this will be a reduced risk compared to non-use of contraception)

- a small number of women will develop functional ovarian cysts
- removal can be complicated if implants are not inserted
- correctly

Contra-indications
- possible pregnancy
- active thromboembolic disorders
- undiagnosed vaginal bleeding
- undiagnosed uterine disorder
- known or suspected cancer of the reproductive organs
- recent trophoblastic disease until elevated hCG levels are back to normal
- acute liver disease

Side-effects

Side-effects are similar to other progestogen-only methods. Prolonged, irregular menstrual bleeding can continue for up to a year, so *must* be fully discussed.

Benign intracranial hypertension has been reported on rare occasions in users of hormonal methods including Norplant. Although a causal relationship has not been established, the diagnosis should be considered if significant episodes of headache or visual disturbance occur. Norplant should be removed if the diagnosis is confirmed.

Periods

Menstrual irregularity and disruption appear to be most common during the first year of use when the progestogen levels are highest.

Planning a pregnancy

Implants can be removed at any point if a pregnancy is wanted. Fertility returns very quickly once the implant is removed.

Use after childbirth

Implants can be inserted from day 21 after childbirth. If inserted after this time, an additional contraceptive method should be used for 7 days. Any long-term effects relating to breast-feeding are not known. However, use of other progestogen-only methods are known to be safe.

Use after a miscarriage or abortion

Implants can be used immediately after an early miscarriage or abortion and are effective immediately.

Operations/ surgery

Progestogen implants need not be removed in the case of major surgery, but in cases of high risk thrombosis, consideration should be given to standard prophylactic measures.

Drug interactions

There are no data on drug interactions and implants. Although not established for non-oral systemically administered contraceptive steroids, the Manufacturer's Summary of Product Characteristics (SPCs) suggests that drugs that affect the combined pill must be presumed to affect implants.

Antibiotics do not reduce the effectiveness of implants or any other progestogen-only method.

Removal of implants

Norplant can be removed at any time, but should be removed within 5 years of insertion. Removal can occur at any time in the menstrual cycle. Loss of contraceptive efficacy is immediate, so women should be appropriately advised. The implant is removed through a small incision using small forceps (eg Mosquito). Removal usually takes 10-30 minutes. Where removal is a problem specialist advice should be sought. Advice can be obtained from the FFPRHC. If the method is to be continued, a new set of rods can be inserted through the same incision but placed in the opposite direction. Removal of Implanon takes about 2-3 minutes using gentle traction.

Future types of implant

Several different types of hormonal implants are now being developed. Most involve fewer rods than Norplant, for example Jadelle (formerly called Norplant 2), and will be effective for different lengths of time. Biodegradable and non-biodegradable implants are being studied. Injectable microspheres and microcapsules are also being developed.

Further reading

Articles

'Norplant: the UK Experience'
Bromham D
ESC Newsletter, 6, 1996, 2-3

'Norplant implants in the UK: first year continuation and removals'
Peers T, Stevens J and Graham J, et al
Contraception, 53, 1996, 345-51

'A 4-year pilot study on the efficacy and safety of Implanon, a single-rod hormonal contraceptive implant, in healthy women in Thailand'
Kiriwat O, Patanayindee A, Koetsawang S, et al
The European Journal of Contraception and Reproductive Health Care 1998, 3, 85-91

The intrauterine system

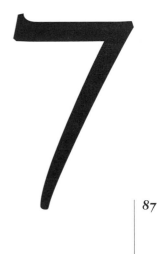

General information

The intrauterine system (IUS) is a levonorgestrel-releasing T-shaped device developed jointly by the Population Council and Leiras. Since the 1970s, research has focused on developing an IUD which releases progestogen. The first such device was trialled in 1977. Progestasert, which delivers progesterone at a rate of 65mcg a day, became available in 1979. Its discontinuation in the UK was primarily for commercial reasons, an uncertainty about an increased risk of ectopic pregnancy and the fact that it had to be replaced annually. Progestasert is available in the United States.

The only IUS currently available in the UK is Mirena. Mirena consists of a T-shaped silastic frame, identical to the Nova-T/Novagard frame. It carries 52mg of levonorgestrel in a cylindrical reservoir attached to the vertical arm of the T. It releases 20mcg of levonorgestrel per 24 hours, through a rate-limiting membrane. It has two monofilament threads for checking and removal.

Mode of action

The IUS works in a number of ways. The effect of levonorgestrel locally suppresses the endometrium, so preventing implantation. In addition, it alters cervical mucus function and utero-tubal fluids which impair sperm migration through the uterus and fallopian tubes. Effects on ovulation vary from anovulation to normal function. After one year most cycles (85 per cent) are ovulatory.

Efficacy

The IUS is very effective with an efficacy rate of over 99 per cent (0.2-0.5 per 100 women failure rate).

Advantages

- highly effective
- immediate fertility return after removal
- reduces menstrual blood loss (it is a recommended method of choice for women with heavy periods)
- reduces dysmenorrhoea
- reduces risk of ectopic pregnancy
- long-acting and independent of intercourse
- reduces PID

Disadvantages   There are very few disadvantages with the IUS:

> ▶ can cause irregular bleeding in the first three months (sometimes longer) of use
> ▶ it has to be fitted
> ▶ sometimes the IUS may be expelled or become displaced
> ▶ some women may develop functional ovarian cysts, but these usually resolve spontaneously
> ▶ there are other rare complications, eg perforation of the uterus/cervix
> ▶ some progestogenic symptoms, such as breast tenderness or acne in early months of use
> ▶ there is a small risk of ectopic pregnancy in the event of IUS failure (any risk is still much less than in women not using contraception)

Contra-indications   For full information see Manufacturer's Summary of Product Characteristics (SPCs).

> ▶ sensitivity to levonorgestrel
> ▶ suspected intrauterine or ectopic pregnancy
> ▶ unexplained uterine or vaginal bleeding
> ▶ current active or recurrent pelvic infection
> ▶ any untreated STIs
> ▶ distorted uterine cavity or cervical abnormalities
> ▶ recent trophoblastic disease until elevated hCG levels are back to normal
> ▶ past history of attack of bacterial endocarditis or severe infection
> ▶ severe arterial disease
> ▶ heart valve replacement – will require specialist advice
> ▶ active liver disease

Note: the IUS has not been shown to be effective as a postcoital intrauterine contraceptive.

Administration   The IUS should only be fitted by doctors trained in fitting and inserting IUDs. The selection of clients, and the training and skill of insertion are critical to the success of the IUS and will affect how the IUS is accepted and used.

The insertion of the IUS is almost identical to that of the Nova-T. However, the insertion tube is wider (4.8mm rather than 3.7mm). All women should be offered pre-medication. This can be oral analgesia or local anaesthesia to the cervix.

With the rising incidence of some STIs, notably Chlamydia trachomatis, a good sexual history must be taken and consideration should be given to screening for infection before IUS insertion. The taking of vaginal and endocervical microbiological swabs (and treatment where necessary) will reduce the incidence of post-fitting sepsis.

Resuscitation facilities should be available and known about when the IUS is fitted (see IUDs, 'Resuscitation procedures', page 98).

Timing of insertion

Ideally, the IUS should be fitted within the first 7 days of a period. If fitted during this time it is effective immediately. If fitted after this time, an additional contraceptive method should be used for 7 days. To minimise expulsion, it is useful to avoid insertion on the 'heaviest' days of a woman's period.

Using the IUS after childbirth

The IUS can be fitted at about 6 weeks after a vaginal delivery in women who are not breast-feeding. After Caesarian delivery, the normal practice is to defer insertion for at least 8 weeks after childbirth.

Using the IUS after a miscarriage or abortion

The IUS may be fitted immediately after a first trimester miscarriage or abortion and is effective immediately.

Instructions for use

Once the IUS is fitted, a woman needs to be taught to feel the IUS threads which come through the cervix. This enables her to check that the IUS is in place. This should be done regularly each month after the end of a period. Where bleeding is irregular, it should be done at a regular monthly interval. If the threads cannot be felt, or if the plastic end of the IUS can be felt, this should be investigated immediately as it might mean the IUS is being expelled, possible perforation or that the threads have been withdrawn up into the uterus. The IUS should not be relied on as a contraceptive until this has been investigated.

Duration of use The IUS is licensed in the UK for 5 years.

Side-effects

Periods and bleeding problems
In the first three months (or longer) bleeding tends to be irregular and commonly results in semi-continuous spotting. Women need to be informed about this and advised that this pattern normally improves. Long-term use results in reduced blood loss (75-97 per cent reduction) with light monthly bleeds, spotting or amenorrhoea in about 20 per cent of women.

Other hormonal effects
Other transient hormonal side-effects can include breast tenderness, headache and acne. Functional ovarian cysts may occur; these usually resolve spontaneously and are not harmful. Lower abdominal pain, back pain, vaginal discharge, depression and nausea have been noted in a small minority of women.

Actinomyces-like organisms (ALOs) in cervical smears
See IUDs, 'ALOs in cervical smears', page 101.

Perforation and expulsion
See IUDs, 'Perforation', page 102 and 'Expulsion', page 102.

Missing or lost threads
See IUDs, 'Missing or lost threads', page 102.

Planning a pregnancy Women who want to become pregnant should be advised that fertility usually returns to normal very rapidly after removal. All known pregnancies following IUS discontinuation have been normal.

Drug interactions

The Manufacturer's Summary of Product Characteristics (SPCs) does not list any drugs that interact to reduce the efficacy of the IUS. It should be noted that enzyme inducing drugs lower progestogen levels in the blood, but as the IUS action is primarily on the endometrium this interaction is not considered significant for the IUS.

Follow-up

Regular check-ups are advised. After the insertion of the IUS a woman should be seen within the first few weeks, or sooner if there is a problem, then after six months and then yearly.

Removal

The IUS is usually removed during a period. If it is removed during the menstrual cycle, an additional contraceptive method needs to be used for 7 days prior to removal if pregnancy is to be avoided.

Intrauterine contraceptive devices

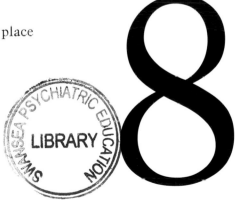

General information

Intrauterine contraceptive devices (IUDs) are small polyethylene and copper devices (some with silver cores) or polymer devices impregnated with medication (such as levonorgestrel-releasing IUDs, see previous chapter on the IUS). These come in varying shapes and sizes and are inserted into the uterus. Newer devices are flexible and frameless, such as GyneFix. Barium sulphate in the polyethylene makes the devices radio-opaque so they can be located, if necessary, by X-ray or ultrasound. Plastic IUDs (Lippes Loop and Saf-t-Coil) are no longer available in the UK, but may still be worn by some women. All devices have monofilament threads for removal and to allow women to check regularly that the IUD is in position. They are effective for a number of years. See 'Duration of use', page 99.

IUDs are under-utilised and are associated with unrealistic negative perceptions which limit their use. Importantly, the following should be taken note of:

▶ IUDs prevent fertilisation and do not cause abortion
▶ nulliparous women may be good candidates if properly selected and an appropriate IUD used
▶ the risk of PID is not increased if the IUD is restricted to women with low risk for STIs
▶ proper IUD fitting and provision requires training which includes current scientific information, insertion practice and information/advice-giving techniques

Mode of action

The antifertility effect of IUDs appears to be the result of a variety of mechanisms, the main effect being to prevent fertilisation. They do not cause abortion. WHO has concluded:

'It is unlikely that the contraceptive efficacy of IUDs results, mainly or exclusively, from their capacity to interfere with implantation; it is more probable that they exert their antifertility effects beyond the uterus and interfere with steps in the reproductive process that take place before the ova reach the uterine cavity. It is likely

*that the uterine and tubal fluids that are altered in the
presence of an IUD impair the viability of the gametes,
thus reducing their chances of union and impeding
fertilization. Copper ions released by an IUD probably
potentiate these effects.'*

All IUDs cause a foreign body reaction in the endometrium,
with increased numbers of leucocytes. Hormone-releasing
IUDs work in a similar way to other progestogen-only
preparations, and may inhibit ovulation, in addition to
the normal action of IUDs (see 'The IUS', page 87).

Table 7 gives a description of IUDs available in the UK.

Efficacy

IUDs are highly effective methods and benefit from no
'user' failures. Today's modern IUDs have very low failure
rates compared to the earlier first generation (plastic only)
and second generation IUDs. The general effectiveness
of IUDs ranges from between 98 to almost 100 per cent.
The newer third generation devices with larger surface
areas of copper such as the Gyne-T 380 (previously called
Ortho Gyne-T 380S) have failure rates of less than 1 per
100 after one year of use. After the first year of use, most
devices have a lower failure rate.

Advantages

▶ provides long-term, highly effective, reversible
  contraception
▶ effective immediately after fitting
▶ non-intercourse related
▶ requires no daily action or remembering
▶ very low morbidity

Disadvantages

▶ may cause menstrual irregularities with inter-menstrual
  bleeding and spotting
▶ periods may be heavier, longer and more painful,
  especially at first
▶ sometimes the IUD may be expelled or become displaced
▶ some women develop a pelvic infection: the risk appears
  to be highest in the first few weeks after insertion.
▶ Pelvic infection is more likely in younger and nulliparous

women, and in women who are at risk of STIs

▶ there are other extremely rare complications, eg perforation

▶ there is a risk of ectopic pregnancy in the event of IUD failure (there is less risk with IUDs releasing copper with a surface area of more than 300mm^2; any risk is still less than in women not using contraception)

Contra-indications

For full information see Manufacturer's Summary of Product Characteristics (SPCs).

▶ known or suspected intrauterine or ectopic pregnancy
▶ any unexplained uterine or vaginal bleeding
▶ menorrhagia (heavy bleeding)
▶ present PID (or possible past infection)
▶ any untreated STI
▶ past history of bacterial endocarditis or severe infection
▶ established immunosuppression
▶ heart valve replacement – will require specialist advice
▶ distorted uterine cavity or cervical abnormalities
▶ previous ectopic pregnancy, or high risk for ectopic pregnancy (eg tubal surgery)
▶ copper allergy (this is rare)
▶ women who are at risk of getting an STI

Administration

IUDs should only be fitted by doctors trained in fitting and inserting IUDs. The selection of clients, the timing and skill of insertion and the choice of device is critical to the success of IUDs and will affect how an IUD is accepted, as well as determine its continuation of use.

With the rising incidence of some STIs, notably Chlamydia trachomatis, a good sexual history must be taken. It is increasingly understood to be good practice to screen for infection before IUD insertion. Taking appropriate microbiological samples and offering treatment (including contact tracing, where necessary) could be expected to reduce the incidence of post-fitting sepsis.

Resuscitation procedures

- resuscitation facilities should be available and known about
- IUD insertion should always be carried out in a relaxed and unhurried atmosphere
- at any sign of a vasovagal attack, insertion needs to be discontinued. The woman should be kept lying down with her head lowered and her legs well elevated
- maintain a clear airway; loosen clothing around the neck
- a Lederal mask or other appropriate appliance should always be available
- avoid over-treatment
- where persistent bradycardia is evident, atropine may be given in a dose of 0.6mg iv
- oxygen if available can be given using an Ambu bag

Timing of insertion

IUDs may be inserted up to day 19 of a 28-day menstrual cycle. The usual time is at the end of a period, when the bleeding is less, minimising the risk of expulsion, and when it is also obvious that a woman is not pregnant.

Using the IUD after childbirth

In the UK, IUDs are not normally fitted immediately after childbirth as there tends to be a higher risk of expulsion. Postpartum IUD insertion usually occurs at about 6 weeks after vaginal delivery. However, immediate post-delivery insertion can be carried out (if there are no contraindications) in skilled hands providing a woman is not breast-feeding. Breast-feeding may increase the risk of perforation. After Caesarian delivery, the normal practice is to defer insertion for at least 8 weeks after birth.

Using the IUD after a miscarriage or abortion

An IUD can be inserted immediately after an early (first trimester) abortion or miscarriage and is effective immediately. If it is not inserted immediately, it should be fitted 2 to 4 weeks later.

Using the IUD after unprotected intercourse

The IUD can be used as a postcoital contraceptive within 5 days of unprotected intercourse or in good faith up to 5 days after the earliest calculation of ovulation (see 'Postcoital contraception', page 149).

Table 7 IUDs available in the UK

Type	Appearance	Manufacturer's recommended life span
Gyne-T 380 Janssen-Cilag	Copper wire on T-shaped polyethylene carrier and copper on vertical section (320mm^2) and copper collars (30mm^2) on each horizontal arm Two monofilament threads	10 years*
Nova-T 380 Schering HC	Copper wires on silver core on T-shape and polyethylene carrier with two monofilament threads Surface area of copper – 380mm^2	5 years*
Nova-T Schering HC	Copper wire with silver core on T-shaped polyethylene carrier with two monofilament threads Surface area of copper – 200mm^2	5 years*
GyneFix Contrel Europe	Copper wire on a non-biodegradable thread on which 6 copper tubes are threaded. The upper and lower tubes are crimped onto the thread to keep tubes in place. The upper extemity of the thread has a knot which serves as an anchor into the fundus. Surface area of copper – 330mm^2	5 years*
Multiload Cu375 Organon	Copper wire on polyethylene carrier with flexible U-shaped side arms with two monofilament threads Surface area of copper – 375mm^2	5 years*
Multiload Cu250 Organon	Copper wire on polyethylene carrier with flexible U-shaped side arms with two monofilament threads Surface area of copper – 250mm^2	3 years*
Multiload Cu250 Short Organon	Copper wire on polyethylene carrier with flexible U-shaped side arms with two monofilament threads Surface area of copper – 250mm^2	3 years*
Flexi-T 300 Prosan International	Copper wire on a flexible T-shaped polyethylene carrier with a single monofilament thread Surface area of copper – 300mm^2	5 years*

*See 'Duration of use' on page 99

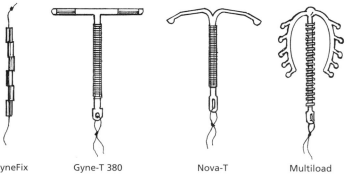

GyneFix   Gyne-T 380   Nova-T   Multiload

Note
These illustrations are smaller than lifesize

An IUD in place

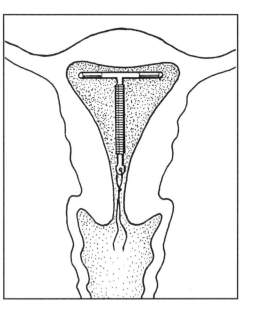

Instructions for use

Once the IUD is fitted, a woman should be taught to feel the IUD threads which come through the cervix. This enables a woman to check that her IUD is in place. This should be done regularly each month after the end of a period. If the strings cannot be felt, or if the plastic end of the IUD can be felt, this should be investigated immediately, as this might mean the IUD is being expelled, possible perforation, or that the threads have been withdrawn up into the uterus. The IUD should not be relied on as a contraceptive until this has been investigated.

Any continued bleeding, pain or unusual vaginal discharge should be checked out by vaginal examination.

Duration of use

Modern copper IUDs have varying life spans of 3 to 10 years, depending on the type of IUD. These differ from country to country and tend to be the minimum lifespans. Extensive clinical research shows that for many devices the lifespan exceeds the manufacturer's recommendations. The Medical Advisory Committees of the **fpa** and the FFPRHC recommend that for routine management modern third generation copper-bearing IUDs may be left in place for at least 5 years. IUDs inserted after the age of 40 can be left in until the menopause. Plastic IUDs still in situ can be left in until the menopause in the absence of any problems.

Side-effects

Periods and bleeding problems

The occurrence of irregular bleeding or heavier and longer periods, particularly in the first couple of months, can be one of the main problems of IUDs for some women. Bleeding and some discomfort in the first couple of days after insertion is quite normal. Any pain (similar to period pains) can be controlled by simple analgesics. Any unusual bleeding, pain or discharge should always be investigated.

Pelvic infection

Pelvic inflammatory disease (PID) is the general term for infection of the upper genital tract, including the uterus, fallopian tubes and ovaries. There is extensive research on the association between use of IUDs and PID. Much of it is inconclusive, and there needs to be a recognition that PID is caused by people, not devices. However, it is generally considered that the overall risk of PID in IUD users is in the range of 1.5 to 2.6. Risks appear to be highest in the first 3 weeks after IUD insertion. The main factors that increase the risk of getting PID are parity, age and sexual activity of the woman and her partner(s).

Symptoms of infection may include pain during or after intercourse, unusual vaginal discharge, lower abdominal or back pain or irregular bleeding. Immediate treatment is necessary to minimise any damage to the reproductive tract.

Actinomyces-like organisms (ALOs) in cervical smears

New recommendations on ALOs were produced by FFPRHC in 1998. A woman whose smear shows the presence of ALOs should have an abdominal and pelvic examination and be asked about the symptoms of pelvic actinomycosis. These include:

- intermenstrual bleeding
- pelvic pain
- deep dyspareunia
- dysuria

With such symptoms of pelvic inflammatory disease, in the presence of ALOs, the IUD should be removed at an appropriate time. The IUD should be sent for culture.

Where ALOs occur in cervical smears in an *asymptomatic* woman, the recommended advice involves choosing between two courses of action: either to leave the device in place or take it out. Good case notes are essential.

Leaving the IUD in place:
- the woman should be seen and a careful history taken; she should be examined and fully counselled about her options and potential risks and symptoms
- finding ALOs in cervical smears does not necessitate the removal of an IUD in the absence of symptoms
- the IUD can be left in provided careful follow-up can be maintained every 6 months and her GP contacted if she fails to attend. To leave the IUD in place, or not, should be the woman's decision after full discussion
- careful follow-up is essential and must include specific instructions to warn about symptoms such as pain, dyspareunia, excessive vaginal discharge and fever, which should lead her to seek *immediate* medical advice
- cervical smears should be repeated as indicated by the National Screening Programme or locally agreed cervical screening guidelines

Taking the IUD out:
- the IUD can be removed and, where appropriate, a new one inserted on the same occasion, ensuring ongoing contraception
- a cervical smear should be repeated in 3 to 6 months and thereafter, as indicated by the findings and cervical screening guidelines

Management in the presence of symptoms or signs (notably pelvic tenderness) should be proactive with the removal and microbiological investigation of the IUD. Endometrial biopsy should be carried out involving histological and bacteriological analysis. Long-term antibiotic treatment should be given as indicated. Future use of the IUD is contraindicated.

Further guidelines are available from the FFPRHC.

Perforation

Perforation where the IUD penetrates through the cervix or the uterus is uncommon (the risk is about 1 in 1,000 insertions). This may happen at insertion, or be diagnosed later. Any loss of threads, or pain or discomfort either after insertion or later should always be checked immediately to rule out perforation or any other problem.

Expulsion

This problem relates to all IUD types. The risk is greatest in the first 3 months after insertion. Expulsion is more common in nulliparous women. Women should be encouraged to check the IUD threads regularly, once a month, after the end of each period.

Missing or lost threads

If the threads cannot be felt during a monthly check the woman should be advised to return to her doctor, and advised not to rely on her IUD until this has been checked. An additional contraceptive method should be used during this time. Missing threads may indicate pregnancy, or that the device has been expelled, possible perforation or that the threads have been withdrawn up into the uterus, or that the IUD has moved. There are various ways this can be checked, all requiring a skilled practitioner or specialist centre.

Pregnancy with an IUD in place

Any suspected pregnancy should be investigated immediately. A pregnancy may be extrauterine or intrauterine. Extrauterine pregnancy (ectopic pregnancy) is a serious problem, and requires immediate referral. An ectopic pregnancy may be associated with a light, scanty or missed period, with or without lower abdominal pain.

Intrauterine pregnancy with an IUD in place may go successfully to term or miscarry. Where possible, if the choice is to continue with the pregnancy, the IUD should be removed. Removal of the IUD should be attempted only if the pregnancy is less than 12 weeks advanced, and the threads are easily visible and offer no resistance to removal. (In the absence of visible threads, ultrasound can be used.) The risk of miscarriage is higher (over 50 per cent) if the IUD is left in place, than if it is removed (where the miscarriage rate is about 20 per cent). There is no evidence of any abnormality in the baby if the pregnancy goes to term. The IUD is usually expelled with the afterbirth as it is positioned outside the gestational sac containing the baby. If it is not expelled with the placenta, location of the device is essential. It should not be assumed that it was expelled at an earlier time.

Drug interactions

Antibiotic therapy does not interfere with copper IUDs. Reports that the use of anti-inflammatory drugs such as aspirin and corticosteroids increases the failure rate of IUDs have not been confirmed, but corticosteroid therapy may increase the susceptibility to infection.

Diathermy

Short wave diathermy is not a contraindication in IUD users, but is considered a theoretical risk and so caution is advised. Copper bearing or inert IUDs can be left in situ during an MRI scan.

Follow-up

Regular check-ups are advised. After insertion of the IUD a woman should be seen within the first few weeks or sooner if there is a problem, then after 6 months, and then yearly. If a woman wishes to become pregnant, the IUD is easily removed, usually during a period. There is no detrimental effect on fertility.

Removal

The IUD is usually removed during a period. If it is removed during the menstrual cycle, an additional contraceptive method needs to be used for 7 days prior to removal if pregnancy is to be avoided.

New IUDs

New IUDs being researched include modified designs, such as flexible and frameless IUDs, to help reduce expulsion and other side-effects associated with current IUDs.

Further reading

Books

Mechanism of action, safety and efficacy of intrauterine devices
Technical Report Series 753
WHO, 1987

Contraception – your questions answered
Guillebaud J
2nd edn, Churchill Livingstone, 1993 (revised 1994)
Chapter 6: Intrauterine devices

Handbook of family planning and reproductive health care
Loudon N, Glasier A and Gebbie A (eds)
3rd edn, Churchill Livingstone, 1995
Chapter 5: Intrauterine contraceptive devices, Drife J

Population Reports: IUDs – an update
Series B No 6, December 1995
Population Information Program
Johns Hopkins School of Public Health

Articles
'New insights into the mode of action of intrauterine devices'
Alvarez F, Brache V and Fernandez E, et al
Fertility and Sterility, 49, 1988, 768-73

'Intrauterine devices and pelvic inflammatory disease: an international perspective'
Farley T M M, Rosenberg M J and Rowe P J, et al
The Lancet, 339, 1992, 785-88

'Long-term use of contraceptive uterine devices – a statement from the Medical Advisory Committee of the **fpa** and NAFPD'
Newton J and Tacchi D
The Lancet, 335, 1990, 1322-23

'Recommendations for clinical practice: actinomyces-like organisms and intrauterine contraceptives'
The Clinical and Scientific Committee of the FFPRHC
British Journal of Family Planning, 23, 1998, 137-8

Female barrier methods – Diaphragm, cap, female condom

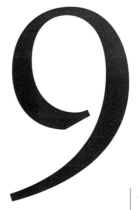

General information

There is now a variety of female barrier methods to choose from. These include diaphragms, caps and female condoms. Diaphragms and caps should always be used with spermicides.

Diaphragms and caps

Diaphragms and caps are available from family planning clinics, family doctors and pharmacies.

Mode of action

They fit into the vagina and cover the cervix to provide a barrier between the egg and sperm, so preventing fertilisation.

Efficacy

When used carefully and correctly with spermicide, diaphragms and caps have an effectiveness rate of 92-96 per cent.

Products available

See Table 8.

Diaphragms

Diaphragms, commonly known as caps, are thin soft latex rubber, dome-shaped devices with a flexible circular ring covered by rubber. They come in different sizes from 55mm to 100mm rising in 5mm steps. They fit into the vagina between the posterior fornix and behind the pubic bone to cover the cervix. The diaphragm is held in place by the vaginal muscles, the tension of the ring and the pubic bone. There are three types of diaphragm.

Flat spring

The rim contains a firm, flat watch-spring metal band and squeezes flat for insertion. These diaphragms are suitable for women with normal vaginas, and are usually offered first. They come in sizes of 55-95mm.

Coil spring

The rim contains a round spiral of coiled metal wire. It is more flexible than the flat spring type. Where a flat spring diaphragm is not suitable, a coil spring should be tried, providing the woman has good vaginal muscle tone. Because they are more flexible they can be more comfortable than the flat spring. They come in sizes of 55-100mm.

Arcing spring

This combines the features of the coil and flat spring diaphragm. It squeezes into an arc for insertion and provides a useful alternative for women who have poor vaginal muscular support, or where the length or the position of the cervix makes fitting of a coil spring or flat spring diaphragm more difficult. It comes in sizes of 60-95mm.

Caps

Caps are smaller than diaphragms. They are made of rubber and fit directly over the cervix. They are held in place mainly by suction and by support from the vaginal wall. They come in different shapes and sizes. Caps are a useful alternative for women who wish to use a barrier method, but cannot use diaphragms. They appear to be used only rarely, in part because many professionals are not trained or confident in fitting them.

Cervical cap (Prentif cavity rim)

This is a thick rim cervical cap. It is a deep, soft cap which is shaped like a thimble, with a firm rim and groove around the inner lip of the rim. This provides the suction. It comes in four sizes ranging from 22mm to 31mm, rising in 3mm steps.

Vault cap (Dumas cap)

This is a semi-circular, shallow, dome-shaped cap, which comes in five sizes 1-5 ranging from 55mm to 75mm, rising in 5mm steps.

Vimule cap

This combines the features of the cervical and vault caps. It is dome-shaped with a thinner splayed rim which adheres to the vaginal walls. It comes in three sizes 1-3 ranging from 42mm to 54mm.

Table 8 Diaphragms and caps

Product & manufacturer	Description	Colour	Size
Diaphragms			
Reflexions Lamberts	Flat spring diaphragm	Opaque, satin finish	55-95mm (rising in 5mm steps)
Ortho Janssen-Cilag	Coil spring diaphragm	Opaque	55-100mm (rising in 5mm steps)
Ortho All Flex Janssen-Cilag	Arcing spring diaphragm	Opaque	60-95mm (rising in 5mm steps)
Caps			
Dumas Lamberts	Vault cap	Opaque, cream	55-75mm (rising in 5mm steps) 1-5 sizes
Prentif Cavity Rim Lamberts	Cervical cap	Opaque, cream	22-31mm (rising in 3mm steps) 1-4 sizes
Vimule Cap Lamberts	Vimule cap	Opaque, cream	42-54mm (rising in 6mm steps) 1-3 sizes

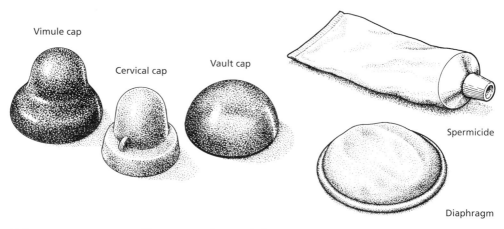

Vimule cap

Cervical cap

Vault cap

Spermicide

Diaphragm

Advantages
► effective with careful use
► can be put in at any convenient time before having sex so it need not interfere with spontaneity
► may protect against cancer of the cervix, some STIs (although not HIV) and PID
► there are no established health risks or systemic side-effects
► under the direct control of the woman

Disadvantages
- ▶ requires thinking ahead so that the diaphragm/cap is in place or readily available
- ▶ requires careful use for it to be effective
- ▶ an increased incidence of cystitis or urinary tract infection in some women using diaphragms
- ▶ must be used with spermicides
- ▶ woman has to be fitted initially to know size and be taught how to use it

Contra-indications
- ▶ very poor muscle tone may be a contraindication for the diaphragm
- ▶ women with a shallow pubic ledge – this applies to the diaphragm only
- ▶ abnormality of the vagina
- ▶ women who are unable to touch their genital area with comfort
- ▶ any irritation, sensitivity or allergy to latex or spermicides
- ▶ a current vaginal, cervical or pelvic infection, or recurrent urinary tract infection
- ▶ past toxic shock syndrome
- ▶ lack of privacy for insertion, removal or care of the diaphragm/cap

Administration

Diaphragms and caps are free on prescription on the NHS. In addition, they can be obtained without prescription by buying them from pharmacies or by mail order (the type and size will need to be known). They should be fitted and their use taught by a trained family planning nurse or doctor. The acceptability of diaphragms and caps is much higher if women are taught by enthusiastic, trained staff. They should always be used with spermicides (see 'Spermicides', page 127).

Instructions for use of diaphragms and caps

The correct size and type for an individual woman can only be determined by vaginal examination. Full instructions should be given on how to use and care for the diaphragm or cap.

Holding a diaphragm

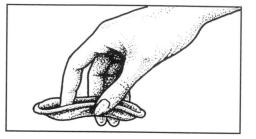

Inserting a diaphragm

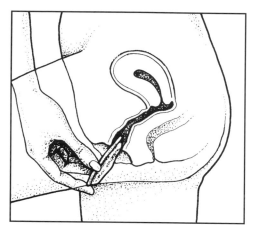

Diaphragm in position

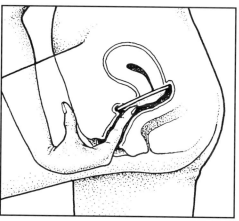

Cap in position

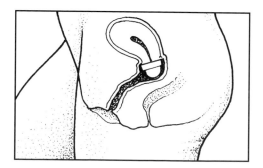

The diaphragm or cap with spermicide can be inserted at any time before having sex. If it is inserted more than 3 hours before intercourse, or if intercourse occurs more than once, additional spermicide should be used without removing the diaphragm or cap. The diaphragm or cap must be left in place for at least 6 hours after intercourse, but should not be left in the vagina for longer than 30 hours (this includes the 6 hours after use). Providing the diaphragm or cap is correctly inserted, neither partner should be able to feel it. If it can be felt or is uncomfortable a woman should have it checked by her doctor or nurse. For some women, the use of an introducer can help with the insertion of a diaphragm.

All oil-based products, such as petroleum jelly, baby oils, bath oils etc, should be avoided with latex products as they cause rapid deterioration of rubber. Oil-based vaginal and rectal medications should also be avoided. After use, the diaphragm or cap should be washed with mild unscented soap, well rinsed and dried carefully. It should be stored in a cool place. It should be checked for any holes or deterioration before each use.

Practice diaphragms or caps are often given to women when they first choose to use these methods. Women must be advised that practice diaphragms or caps should not be relied on as contraceptives. Their purpose is to allow a woman to feel confident about using the method before actively relying on it as a method of birth control. (See 'Decontamination of practice diaphragms and caps', page 114.)

Using diaphragms or caps after childbirth

The diaphragm or cap can be used about 6 weeks after delivery, after vaginal muscle tone is restored. A woman should always be checked for size after childbirth.

Using diaphragms or caps after a miscarriage or abortion

The diaphragm or cap should be checked for size after a miscarriage or abortion as the vagina may change in shape or size.

Duration of use

Diaphragms or caps should be replaced annually, or immediately if any problem such as holes or puckering of the rubber occurs. Discoloration will occur, and is quite normal; it does not affect the latex.

Side-effects

There are few side-effects with these methods.

Irritation

Some women do have increased sensitivity, irritation or allergy to latex or spermicides. It is important that any symptoms are always checked to rule out any pre-existing or new vaginal infection.

Urinary tract infection

There is some indication that some women who use diaphragms develop cystitis and urethritis more frequently than women who use other methods. This may be due to pressure on the urethra, especially if the diaphragm is too big. If this is a recurrent problem, the size of the diaphragm should be carefully checked and, if necessary, one of the smaller cervical caps should be tried.

Toxic shock syndrome

A few cases of toxic shock syndrome have been reported in diaphragm users. Almost all cases have been in women who have worn the diaphragm for more than 30 hours.

Follow-up

Diaphragms and caps should be replaced annually, and checked for size and fitting. They should also be automatically checked after childbirth, abortion or miscarriage or if a woman gains or loses 3kg (7lb) in weight.

Decontamination of practice diaphragms and caps

This is an issue if CSSD is not available.

Where practice diaphragms and caps are used there is a need to ensure effective decontamination practices to prevent transmission of infection between clients. The only currently acceptable methods of decontamination are heat-based. Chemicals are no longer recommended by the Department of Health and should not be used for decontaminating instruments and appliances intended for use in the vagina or cervix.

Sterilisation is the optimal form of decontamination. Sterilisation of diaphragms should be carried out in an autoclave at 121°C. This uses steam under pressure in a controlled and self-monitoring process. At higher temperatures they degrade much more rapidly.

New types of cap

Research is being carried out into producing different kinds of cervical barriers, which may offer methods that are more effective, easier to fit and can be used without spermicides.

The task for researchers is to provide a product that will prevent pregnancy, reduce the risk of some STIs and PID, and at the same time be aesthetic, convenient and effective, and involve minimal medical intervention. Research is still a long way off from that ideal. Three new types of cap are being made available: Lea's Shield, Oves Cap and Femcap.

Lea's Shield

This is a single-size cup-shaped barrier that covers the cervix. It has a U-shaped loop to facilitate removal. Made of silicone, it incorporates a valve in its design to allow draining of cervical secretions and menstrual blood. This valve also creates a surface tension effect allowing the device to fit tightly around the cervix. Studies are ongoing about Lea's Shield acceptability and efficacy. It is available in some parts of Europe and has a CE mark.

Oves Cap

Made of silicone rubber, this disposable thin and flexible cap is designed to be effective for up to 3 days. It is used with spermicide and comes in 3 different sizes: 26mm, 28mm and 30mm. Studies are ongoing about the acceptability and efficacy of the Oves Cap. It has a CE mark.

Femcap

Made of silicone rubber, this device is shaped like a sailor's hat with a wide upturned brim. It fits directly over the cervix and can be worn for up to 48 hours. It has a loop to facilitate removal and is used with spermicide. Femcap comes in two sizes: regular for multiparous women who have had vaginal delivery, small for nulliparous women. Efficacy rates are expected to be comparable with other barrier methods. Randomised comparative trials are being carried out to look at acceptability and efficacy.

Female condom

General information

The female condom is a lubricated, loose fitting polyurethane sheath with two flexible rings, which is inserted into the vagina. It lines the vagina and covers some of the vulva. It comes in one size and does not need to be fitted by a health professional. Female condoms are available from family planning clinics, pharmacies, by mail order and from other retail outlets. It has a CE mark.

Mode of action

The female condom acts as a barrier between sperm and egg, so preventing fertilisation.

Efficacy

At present there are no large studies showing ranges of the effectiveness rates. It has an effectiveness rate of 85-95 per cent.

Products available

At present there is only one female condom available in the UK. It is called Femidom (see Table 9). A number of similar products are being researched.

Advantages

- ▶ no known side-effects
- ▶ it acts as both a contraceptive and prophylactic against STIs, including HIV, and may protect against cancer of the cervix and PID
- ▶ effective with careful use
- ▶ under the direct control of the woman

- ▶ can be inserted at any time before having sex
- ▶ does not require additional spermicide
- ▶ can be used with oil-based products
- ▶ compared to male condoms 'feels' more normal for partner
- ▶ polyurethane is stronger than latex
- ▶ does not need male erection before use

Disadvantages
- ▶ requires thought before use
- ▶ not so discreetly disposable as male condoms
- ▶ requires careful insertion and use for it to be effective
- ▶ can interrupt sex
- ▶ can get pushed into the vagina by penis during sex
- ▶ not widely available from family planning clinics or GPs

Contra-indications
- ▶ women who are unable to touch their genital area with comfort
- ▶ women with a pre-existing vaginal or cervical infection

Instructions for use

If obtained from a family planning clinic, a nurse or doctor can provide instructions on how to use the female condom. If bought at a pharmacy, full instructions are available with the packet. Each female condom is individually packaged. The condom is inserted into the vagina using the inner ring as a guide. The condom should be pushed up behind the pubic bone. The inner ring, as well as acting as a guide, keeps it in place. The outer ring lies flat against the body covering the vulva and helps prevent the condom from being drawn down into the vagina during intercourse. When correctly in place, the condom should loosely line the vagina and feel comfortable. It can be inserted any time before having sex. As with all barrier methods, there should be no genital contact before or after use. Care needs to be taken that the penis is not inserted between the outside of the condom and the vaginal wall. The condom should be used only once. Additional spermicides or lubricants of any type can be used (unlike with latex products).

Future methods

New types of female condoms are being studied to provide a variety of products for women.

Further reading

Books

Contraception – your questions answered
Guillebaud J
2nd edn, Churchill Livingstone, 1993 (revised 1994)
Chapter 3: Vaginal methods of contraception

Handbook of family planning and reproductive health care
Loudon N, Glasier A and Gebbie A (eds)
3rd edn, Churchill Livingstone, 1995
Chapter 6: Barrier methods, Gebbie A

Barrier contraceptives: current status and future prospects
Mauck C, Cordero M and Gabelnick H, et al
Wiley-Liss, 1994

Resource

'Sterilisation, disinfection and cleaning of medical equipment – guidance on decontamination'
Medical Devices Agency, 1996

Article

'The contraceptive efficacy of the diaphragm and cervical caps used in conjunction with a spermicide – a fresh look at the evidence'
Bounds W
British Journal of Family Planning, 20, 1994, 84-87

Letter

'Decontamination of practice diaphragms and caps'
Bounds W
British Journal of Family Planning, 22, 1996, 160

Male barrier methods –
Male condom

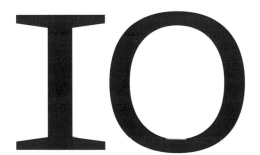

General information

The male condom is one of the oldest methods of family planning and, apart from vasectomy (male sterilisation), it is the only reliable method a man can use. Male condoms are made of natural latex or polyurethane. Condoms are available free from family planning clinics. They are not generally available from family doctors. They can be bought from a variety of sources: pharmacies, retail outlets, by mail order and from garages and vending machines.

Mode of action

The male condom, which fits over the erect penis, acts as a barrier between egg and sperm, so preventing fertilisation.

Efficacy

Male condoms, when used carefully and consistently, are highly effective in preventing both pregnancy and STIs, including HIV. Their general effectiveness ranges from about 85-98 per cent.

Main products available

See Tables 9 and 10.

The **fpa** only recommends condoms which are certified to British Standards Institution (BSI) specification (BS EN 600). Products that have passed these standards are recognised by the Kitemark. The BSI Kitemark scheme of product quality certification requires manufacturers to satisfy the BSI that the entire manufacturing system from raw materials to goods leaving the premises complies with the recognised standard of good manufacturing practice. The use of the Kitemark illustrates a reliable quality product. Currently there is no BSI standard for polyurethane male condoms.

As from 14 June 1998 it is illegal to manufacture condoms for sale anywhere in European Union countries without a government granted CE mark. The CE mark is not a replacement for the Kitemark. The CE marking that appears on the medical device or on its packaging means that the device 'satisfies the requirements essential for it to be fit for its intended purpose' ie that it is medically safe and does not hurt the user by, for example, releasing harmful substances or disintegrating during use. CE marking is not a guarantee of a condom, diaphragm or cap's effectiveness during actual use against pregnancy or disease. The BS EN 600 is the new European Standard and has been adopted by BSI.

Condoms come in a variety of types: latex, polyurethane, unlubricated, lubricated with silicone or spermicide, coloured, ribbed, teat-ended, plain-ended, shaped, non-flavoured or flavoured. Spermicidally lubricated condoms in the UK contain Nonoxynol-9.

Advantages
- no side-effects (unless sensitive to the latex or Nonoxynol 9)
- very effective with careful use
- easy to obtain and use
- the man can take the responsibility for birth control
- can protect either partner against some STIs, including HIV
- may protect the woman against cancer of the cervix and PID
- requires no medical supervision

Disadvantages
- requires forward planning each time
- needs to be used carefully to be effective
- possible loss of sensitivity during intercourse
- may interrupt sex, although putting on the condom can be enjoyed as part of foreplay
- can break or slip off
- needs to be disposed of carefully
- latex condoms should not be used with oil-based products

Contra-indications
- any allergy, irritation or sensitivity to latex or spermicide
- men unable to maintain erection during intercourse

Instructions for use

Where male condoms are provided through community family planning clinics, GUM clinics or through the primary health care team, family planning nurses or doctors can advise on correct usage of the condom.

Full instructions also come with packets if obtained elsewhere.

Like all barrier methods, condoms must be used before any genital contact. To use the condom, the closed or teat end of the condom is squeezed to expel any air and leave about a centimetre to receive the ejaculated semen. It is then rolled down over the full length of the erect penis. After ejaculation the condom should be carefully removed holding it firmly at the rim as the penis is withdrawn.

Male condoms should be used only once. The expiry date on the packet should be checked and all oil-based products should be avoided with latex products. Certain vaginal and rectal medications should also be avoided.

Additional spermicide products of any type can be used if required.

Skin condoms are available to buy, but they are not BSI Kitemarked and are not recommended by the **fpa** for contraception or prophylaxis.

Polyurethane condoms are considered to have some advantages over latex condoms, such as a longer shelf life, possible improved sensation during sexual intercourse, compatibility with oil-based products and lack of latex smell.

It is generally assumed that everyone knows how to use condoms, but this is not the case. Health professionals are in an ideal position to help with any concerns or queries.

Side-effects

There are no adverse side-effects of male condoms except possible sensitivity, irritation or allergy to the latex or spermicide. If this is a problem a non-spermicidally lubricated or hypoallergenic type is recommended. Many condoms are now produced from hypoallergenic latex. Polyurethane condoms are also a choice.

Table 9 Non-latex condoms, no BSI standard available

Manufacturer & product	Presentation
LRC Products (Durex)	
Non-spermicidally lubricated	
Avanti	polyurethane, larger/looser, lightweight, odourless, unaffected by oil-based lubricants, teat end
Condomi Health (UK)	
Non-spermicidally lubricated	
E-Z-on	polyurethane, larger/looser, lightweight, odourless, unaffected by oil-based lubricants, with donning device, teat end
Female Health Company Limited (Femidom)	
Femidom	polyurethane, female condom, gently lines the vagina like a second skin and also covers some of the vulva, odourless, unaffected by oil-based lubricants

Future types of condom

Research is currently being carried out into different varieties of condoms, including some made of different kinds of polymers, to improve sensitivity and user acceptability. Improvements in design include changes in shape, loose-fitting condoms instead of snug fit designs, and improved packaging to ensure 'right way on' use.

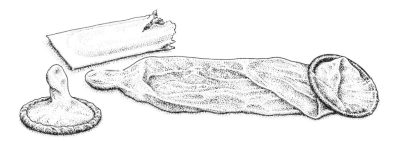

Table 10 Main varieties of Kitemarked condoms available in the UK

Manufacturer & product	Presentation
LRC Products (Durex)	
All produced from hypoallergenic latex	
Spermicidally lubricated	
Elite	transparent, straight-sided, lightweight, extra lubricant, teat end
Fetherlight	transparent, straight-sided, ultra-thin, teat end
Extra Safe	coral coloured, anatomically-shaped, teat end
Safe Play	transparent, straight-sided, teat end
Non-spermicidally lubricated	
Select	selection of coloured and flavoured, straight-sided, teat end
Ultra Strong	transparent, straight-sided, stronger/thicker, plain end
Gossamer	transparent, straight-sided, teat end
Comfort	transparent, anatomically-shaped, larger/looser, teat end
Ribbed	coral coloured, straight-sided, ribbed surface, teat end
Mates Healthcare (Mates)	
Spermicidally lubricated	
Natural	transparent, anatomically-shaped, teat end
Ultrasafe	transparent, anatomically-shaped, teat end
Ribbed	transparent, straight-sided, ribbed surface, teat end
Conform	transparent, anatomically-shaped, smaller/tighter, teat end
Variety	selection of coloured, ribbed and natural; straight-sided, natural, anatomically-shaped, all teat end
Sensitive	transparent, anatomically-shaped, lightweight, teat end
Choices	selection of Natural, Ultrasafe and Conform; all transparent, anatomically-shaped, teat end
Non-spermicidally lubricated	
Superstrong	transparent, straight-sided, stronger/thicker, teat end
Intensity	transparent, straight-sided, studded surface, teat end
Original	transparent, straight-sided, teat end

Manufacturer & product	Presentation
Safex Supplies (Safex)	
Spermicidally lubricated	
Natural	transparent, straight-sided, teat end
Sensitive	transparent, straight-sided, lightweight, teat end
Fantasy Ribbed	transparent, anatomically-shaped, ribbed surface, teat end
Non-spermicidally lubricated	
Safe Guard Forte	transparent, straight-sided, stronger/thicker, teat end
Natural Non-Spermicidal	transparent, straight-sided, teat end
Condomi Health (UK)	
Spermicidally lubricated	
Super Safe	transparent, anatomically-shaped, teat end
Non-spermicidally lubricated	
Red Ribbon	transparent, straight-sided, stronger/thicker, plain end
Strong	transparent, straight-sided, stronger/thicker, teat end
Nature	transparent, straight-sided, teat end
Fruit	coloured, straight-sided, scented, teat end
XXL	transparent, straight-sided, larger/looser, teat end
Noppy	transparent, straight-sided, studded surface, teat end
Mix	selection of Nature, XXL and Noppy, all straight-sided, XXL larger/looser, Noppy studded surface, all teat end
Forget Me Not (produced for FP Sales Ltd)	transparent, straight-sided, teat end

Further reading

Books

Barrier contraceptives: current status and future prospects
Mauck C, Cordero M and Gabelnick H, et al
Wiley-Liss, 1994

Handbook of family planning and reproductive health care
Loudon N, Glasier A and Gebbie A (eds)
3rd edn, Churchill Livingstone, 1995
Chapter 6: Barrier methods, Gebbie A

Article

'The male polyurethane condom: a review of current knowledge'
Rosenberg M J, Waugh M S and Soloman H M, et al
Contraception, 53, 1996, 141-146

'Breakage and acceptability of a polyurethane condom: a randomised controlled study'
Frezieres R G, Walsh T L and Nelson A, et al
Family Planning Perspectives, 30, 1998, 73-78

Spermicides

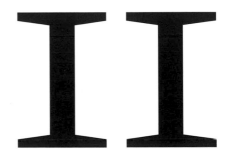

General information

Spermicides are chemical compounds in the form of aerosol foams, jellies, creams, films or pessaries that are inserted into the vagina prior to intercourse. They are not an effective contraceptive method when used alone but, importantly, better than no method at all and are generally used with barrier methods (except for use by women during the menopause when fertility is low).

Mode of action

The main chemical constituent in UK spermicide preparations is Nonoxynol-9 in an inert base. Spermicides kill sperm mainly by altering the integrity of the sperm cell membrane. In addition, the vaginal pH is altered providing an inhospitable environment for sperm.

Products available

See Table 11.

Advantages

▶ no serious side-effects
▶ easily available and simple to use
▶ provides lubrication
▶ provides some protection against STIs, including HIV
▶ enhances efficacy of barrier methods

Disadvantages

▶ should not be used as sole contraceptive
▶ possible sensitivity, irritation or allergy
▶ can be perceived as messy

Instructions for use

All spermicide products should be used in conjunction with barrier methods. Use and efficacy of spermicides vary according to the type used. Type of spermicide, perfume and lubricating properties may influence choice. Applicators for some creams, jellies and foams are available.

Side-effects

There are few side-effects due to spermicides. Allergy is rare; sensitivity or irritation is more common. If sensitivity or irritation occur, another brand (with a different pH) should be tried. Any existing vaginal infection should be checked out as this can be exacerbated by spermicide use. Research shows no adverse effects on the fetus if spermicides are inadvertently used during pregnancy.

Manufacture of the contraceptive vaginal sponge (marketed under the name Today) has been discontinued. Other contraceptive sponges are being researched to look at ways of improving efficacy and reducing STIs and preventing pregnancy.

Future methods   Research is being carried out into the development of more effective, longer-acting spermicides with different base materials.

Entirely new compounds are being explored to act as spermicides, microbiocides and vaginal virucides. Researchers are examining ways to improve acceptability, including evaluation of systems to deliver them. These include sponges, vaginal rings, vaginal pessaries, vaginal tablets and other carriers.

Table 11 Spermicide products

Products & manufacturer/ distributor	Chemical constituents	pH	Presentation
Foam supplied in aerosol containers, with or without an applicator			
Delfen Foam Janssen-Cilag	Nonoxynol-9, 12.5% in a water miscible base	4.5-5.0	20g with applicator refill 20g
Cream supplied in metal tubes			
Ortho-Creme Janssen-Cilag	Nonoxynol-9, 2% in a water miscible base	6.0	70g *
Jellies supplied in metal tubes			
Duragel LRC	Nonoxynol-9, 2%	6.0-7.0	100g *
Gynol II Janssen-Cilag	Nonoxynol-9, 2% in a water soluble base	4.5-4.7	81g *
Pessaries			
Ortho-Forms Janssen-Cilag	Nonoxynol-9, 5% in a water soluble base	4.0-5.0	15 individually sealed pessaries
Double Check FP Sales	Nonoxynol-9, 6% in a water soluble base	4.5-7.5	10 individually sealed pessaries

*Separate applicator available

Natural family planning/ fertility awareness

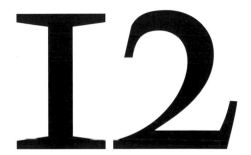

General information

The traditional terms 'rhythm' and 'safe period' to designate family planning based on the detection of ovulation have been replaced over the last decade by the terms 'natural family planning (NFP)' or 'fertility awareness'. NFP methods are based on the recognition of the naturally occurring signs and symptoms of ovulation identifying the fertile and infertile phases of the menstrual cycle in order to plan or prevent a pregnancy. Some of these relate directly to the sexual and reproductive organs, some relate to other systems in the body and on moods and emotions. Nature has equipped women with a highly effective 'built in' fertility system. However, awareness levels of this system are low amongst women.

Fertility awareness involves understanding basic information about fertility and reproduction and being able to apply this knowledge. It provides a woman (and her partner) with knowledge, sensitivity and understanding of the natural rhythms and changes in her body.

Natural family planning methods

There are a number of recognised indicators:

► cycle length
► waking body temperature
► cervical secretions (cervical mucus)
► combining indicators
► fertility devices

How natural family planning methods work

All these methods are intended to help to recognise or predict the timing of ovulation, by identifying the fertile and infertile phases of the menstrual cycle. Ovulation is the result of a complex and delicate sequence of events in the body, which occur 12-16 days *before* a woman's next period. The egg remains capable of being fertilised for up to a maximum of 24 hours and sperm are capable of fertilising an egg for about 3-5 days, sometimes longer, up to 7 days. Because of this the fertile phase is a relatively short time each month.

Cycle length indicator

This involves working out the probability of the fertile time in advance each month based on the calculations of 6 to 12 menstrual cycles. This is no longer recognised as a reliable single indicator of fertility, as it makes no allowance for cycle irregularity, stress, illness, etc.

Temperature indicator

This relies on the measurement of normal changes in body temperature that occur after ovulation. Immediately after ovulation, basal body temperature (BBT – the body's temperature at complete rest) drops slightly and then rises by about 0.2° to 0.4°C. It stays high until just before the next period. The pattern of a low temperature for the first part of the cycle and a higher temperature for the second part is known as a biphasic pattern and can be observed if an accurate record of daily temperature is maintained throughout the cycle.

As a single indicator of fertility, using the temperature method restricts the time in which unprotected sexual intercourse can take place if a pregnancy is not wanted. The efficacy of the temperature method used alone is low as it does not indicate the beginning of the fertile phase. If intercourse is restricted to after ovulation – the second infertile phase of the cycle only, efficacy is improved.

Cervical mucus indicator

This relies on the detection of changes in cervical mucus which occur during the menstrual cycle. By noting the changes between 'infertile' and 'fertile' mucus, ovulation can be predicted and detected.

Cyclic hormonal variations and changes associated with ovulation are directly reflected in cervical mucus. The presence or absence of mucus secretions can be observed by:

▶ sensations of dryness, moistness, slipperiness in the vagina
▶ checking the appearance of the mucus for colour and stretchiness
▶ a combination of these

Directly after a period, when oestrogen levels are low, cervical mucus is scanty and dry; this is known as infertile mucus. As ovulation approaches, changes in the cervical mucus occur. As oestrogen levels rise the cervical mucus increases in volume, fluidity and clarity, with an appearance like raw egg white. This is known as 'fertile' mucus. The last day of fertile mucus is known as the peak mucus day. The peak mucus day corresponds with the peak secretion of oestrogen in the bloodstream, which occurs about one day before the Luteinising Hormone (LH) peak. This precedes ovulation by not more than 48 hours. The infertile phase will begin on the evening of the fourth day after the peak mucus day.

Combining indicators

This combines all the primary and secondary indicators of fertility, and because of this it is also referred to as the multiple index method or double check method. Some women know intuitively whether they are fertile from a number of physical and emotional changes occurring in the two weeks before a period. For example, in addition to primary indicators (such as temperature and mucus), secondary indicators such as changes occurring in the position and softness of the cervix, width of the cervical os, mid-cycle ovulation pain (mittelschmerz), discharge or bleeding, breast sensitivity or mood changes, enable a woman to have a lot of information about her body. Women may experience some or all of these changes. The choice of indicators depends on which signs and symptoms are predominant in each individual woman and the ease with which she can observe them.

Efficacy

Combining more than one fertility indicator is the most effective of the NFP methods. The effectiveness ranges from 80 to 98 per cent.

Changes during the menstrual cycle

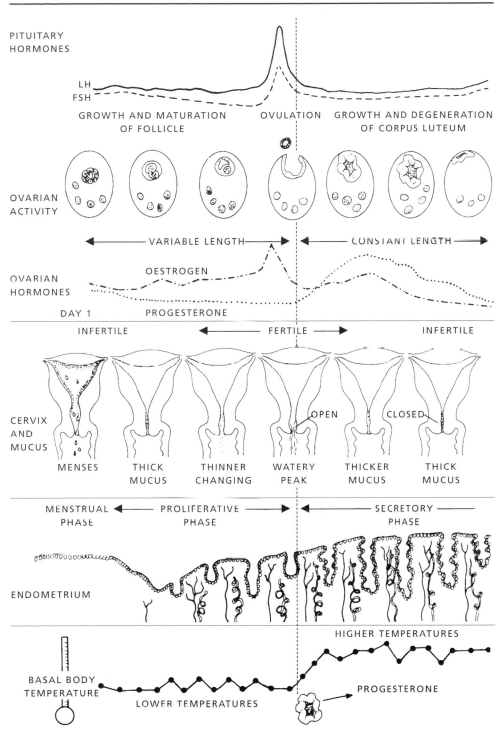

Reproduced with kind permission from Fertility – fertility awareness and natural family planning *by Elizabeth Clubb and Jane Knight, 3rd edn, David & Charles, 1996*

Advantages
- can be used to plan a pregnancy as well as prevent conception
- there are no known physical side-effects
- non-intercourse related method
- couples share responsibility for family planning and may become more aware of how their bodies work
- some couples feel they enjoy intercourse more after abstaining during the fertile time
- no mechanical devices or hormones are used
- it is acceptable to all religions
- once the method has been learnt by the user, no further follow-up (unless wanted) or expense is necessary

Disadvantages
- it requires the commitment of *both* partners
- for successful use of these methods, teaching is required from specially trained NFP teachers
- the methods require careful observation and record keeping, which may take time to learn
- high motivation is required

Fertility devices

Advances in technology and improved understanding of the reproductive processes have led to a number of fertility devices and systems becoming available. These monitor temperature, saliva and urine. To date these have been expensive, not highly effective and not always easy to use.

Although there is a range of fertility devices available, the launch in October 1996 of the Unipath Personal Contraceptive System, Persona, represented a significant advance on other available products. Following more than 15 years of research, the system consists of a small hand-held computerised monitor and urine test sticks. The system detects hormonal changes related to fertility and is able to interpret these changes to indicate where the user is in her menstrual cycle. The system defines the beginning and end of the fertile phase by pinpointing estrone 3 glucoronide (E3G) and LH. Based on sophisticated diagnostic technology, the system contains simple to use test sticks which sample urine on designated days of the menstrual cycle. The electronic monitor reads the test stick and uses a predictive algorithm for interpreting the results and indicating fertility status.

This is shown by a red light for fertile days and green light for non-fertile days. A yellow light indicates that a urine test is required. During the first cycle of use while the monitor receives information about the woman's cycle, 16 test sticks have to be used. This is reduced to 8 test days after this time, providing the guidelines are followed. Because of the accurate monitoring involved, the number of potentially fertile days is considerably reduced compared with other natural method indicators. Based on European trials the manufacturers claim this system to be 94 per cent effective when used according to instructions. Persona is not recommended if pregnancy is not acceptable, if the woman has impaired liver or kidney function or polycystic ovarian syndrome, if she is breast-feeding, when using hormonal methods, if the menstrual cycle is shorter than 23 or longer than 35 days, or if a woman is using tetracycline (the drug itself, not any of its relatives). Persona is not available on the NHS.

New technologies

Research and developments in this area will continue to try and find highly effective products that will enable women to identify the fertile and infertile phases of the menstrual cycle accurately and with ease, to both prevent conception and plan pregnancy.

Sources of help

Unfortunately good NFP teaching is not generally or easily available from community family planning clinics or from primary health care professionals. Specialist help, including a list of trained NFP teachers, can be obtained from Fertility UK (see 'Addresses of useful organisations', page 198, for more details).

Breast-feeding (lactational amenorrhoea method – LAM)

Breast-feeding is and always has been a natural way to space children. It can also provide time for a woman to consider her contraceptive needs for the future following the birth of her baby.

Suckling during breast-feeding induces a reduction in Gonadotrophin Releasing Hormone (GnRH), LH and FSH. This results in amenorrhoea, and stimulation of prolactin secretion and milk production.

Recognising the value of lactational amenorrhoea the 1988 Bellagio Consensus promoted the use of LAM. WHO has confirmed the validity of LAM as an effective contraceptive method offering 98 per cent protection against pregnancy *when* the following conditions exist:

▶ a woman is fully or almost fully breast-feeding (feeding with *no* substitutes and at regular periods on demand, day and night)
▶ the baby is less than six months old
▶ menstruation has not returned

Today, much more recognition should be given to LAM providing the guidelines for its use are strictly adhered to.

Further reading

Books
Fertility – fertility awareness and natural family planning
Clubb E and Knight J
3rd edn, David & Charles, 1996

The manual of natural family planning
Flynn A and Brooks M
3rd edn, Thorsons, 1996

Article
'Consensus statement on the use of breastfeeding as a family planning method'
Bellagio, 1988
Kennedy K I, Rivera R, McNeilly A S
Contraception, 39, 1989, 477-96

Sterilisation

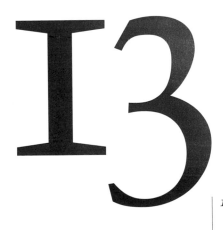

General information

Sterilisation involves cutting, sealing or blocking the fallopian tubes in the woman, or the vasa deferentia in the man, to prevent the egg and sperm meeting. It is usually an elective procedure and should only be considered if the decision is to remain child free or if the family is considered to be complete. Full information and counselling should always be available to ensure that the decision is thought through, and that any worries, problems or questions can be raised and discussed. This must include discussion of any risk of failure. Women and men *must* be advised about information and access to all other long-term reversible methods of contraception as part of the counselling process. This should be properly documented in case notes for any future reference. Ideally the decision to be sterilised should not be made at emotional times such as directly after childbirth, abortion or miscarriage, or when there is a relationship or personal crisis. If there are any doubts, sterilisation should not be carried out. Research shows a higher incidence of regret in some groups. For this reason additional care must be taken when counselling people under the age of 25, those without children and those not in a relationship. At present both male and female sterilisation are still regarded as irreversible procedures. Although reversals can be carried out, there is no guarantee of success. Consent from a partner for the procedure to be carried out is not required by law.

Female sterilisation

Female sterilisation methods

There are a number of different female sterilisation methods. The fallopian tubes which carry the egg from the ovaries to the womb can be reached either directly or indirectly:

▶ directly through an incision in the abdominal wall by laparotomy or mini-laparotomy
▶ indirectly by laparoscopy, or through the vagina by culdoscopy (this is not commonly used in the UK)

Female sterilisation

1 Fallopian tubes cut

2 Fallopian tubes blocked

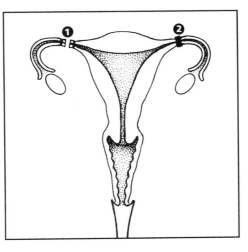

Laparoscopic sterilisation is the most common method today as it is simple, quick and the least invasive. Once the fallopian tubes have been reached they can be blocked by:

► tying and removing a small piece of tube – excision and tubal ligation
► sealing the tubes – cauterisation and diathermy
► blocking the tubes – use of clips (Hulka-Clemens, used less often today, or Filshie) or rings (Falope)

Place of operation

Female sterilisation is carried out either in hospital or in a well-equipped clinic, under a light general anaesthetic, or possibly local anaesthetic. The length of stay varies from a day to a couple of days depending on the method used.

Efficacy

Female sterilisation is effective, with a lifetime failure rate of around 1 in 200. To avoid pregnancy women need to use contraception until their first period after the sterilisation. Research from the US Collaborative Review of Sterilisation (CREST) published in 1996 shows that the risk of recanalisation may be higher than had been previously reported. Sterilisation may fail some years after the procedure and the risk of failure varies by procedure, method and age. The CREST study is unique in its large size, length and follow-up, and the use of life-table analysis of sterilisation procedures. The study emphasises the importance of correct technique in relation to effectiveness of the procedure and to any subsequent ectopic pregnancy risk.

Advantages
▶ highly effective
▶ it is effective immediately
▶ fear of unplanned pregnancy is removed
▶ it is a permanent method

Disadvantages
▶ it involves an operation and anaesthetic
▶ it is not easily reversible

Contra-indications
▶ if there are any marital or relationship problems
▶ uncertainty about the decision to be sterilised
▶ psychiatric illness
▶ physical disability which might increase the risk of the procedure
▶ weight – gross obesity for laparoscopic procedures
▶ certain gynaecological disorders which would make the procedure difficult

Side-effects
There are few serious side-effects with female sterilisation and no serious long-term effects. Ovulation and menstruation continue as before. Some research suggests that some women experience menstrual disturbance and this may relate to age, stopping oral contraception (combined pills), or gynaecological problems such as fibroids.

If pregnancy occurs there is a higher risk of ectopic pregnancy. Any missed, light or scanty period, especially with pain, should be checked to exclude this, and the woman should be examined for pelvic tenderness.

Psychological problems and regret are uncommon where full counselling has been available and where sterilisation is not carried out at a young age (under 25).

Sexual activity and enjoyment should not be affected, and for many it is improved as the fear of unplanned pregnancy is removed. Sexual intercourse can be resumed as soon as a woman feels comfortable. It is important to provide information about the need to continue to use contraception effectively until the sterilisation is carried out and up to the first period *after* sterilisation.

Male sterilisation – Vasectomy

Male sterilisation (vasectomy) involves cutting or blocking the vasa deferentia, the tubes that carry the sperm from the testes to the penis. The vasa are reached via a small incision either in the middle or on each side of the scrotum. A small amount of tube is removed, or cut and sealed by cautery.

Techniques of vasectomy

There are various techniques of vasectomy. In skilled and practised hands side-effects should be minimal. Newer techniques often use very small incisions or punctures. A no-scalpel technique of vasectomy was developed in China in the 1970s by Li Shunqiang. This technique is sometimes known as the Li technique. The no-scalpel technique reaches the vasa via a tiny puncture (approximately 1mm) in the skin rather than an incision. The vasa are drawn through the stretched opening and blocked in the normal way. Sutures are not needed.

The advantages of this technique include a reduction in bleeding, bruising, infection and haematoma compared to the incision technique.

Place of operation

A vasectomy is usually performed under local anaesthetic (sometimes general anaesthetic), as an outpatient procedure in either a hospital or a well-equipped clinic or surgery. It takes about 10-15 minutes. It is safer and simpler than most female sterilisation procedures.

Male sterilisation

1 Vasa deferentia cut

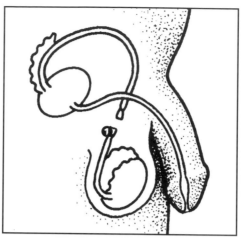

Efficacy

Vasectomy is highly effective, with a lifetime failure rate of about 1 in 2,000. Counselling should always include information about the possibility of failure of vasectomy including late failure due to recanalisation of the vasa deferentia, usually several years after the vasectomy. It is not effective immediately: a vasectomy is considered to be effective only when 2 consecutive negative semen samples have been produced 2 to 4 weeks apart at least 8 weeks after surgery. In some instances sperm clearance can take longer. Until this occurs, an additional contraceptive method must be used at all times.

Failure of vasectomy is a common cause of legal action. Research has shown that fertilisation can occur without a positive semen analysis. This occurs where men intermittently produce small numbers of viable sperm. In these cases paternity needs to be established by DNA analysis. It is therefore important not to jump to conclusions about a partner's sexual activity if pregnancy occurs in the partner of a vasectomised man.

Advantages

▶ simple and easy
▶ it is safe and very effective
▶ fear of unplanned pregnancy is removed
▶ it is a permanent method

Disadvantages	▶ it is not easily reversible
	▶ it is not effective immediately
	▶ it involves a surgical procedure
Contra-indications	▶ certain urological problems
	▶ any marital or relationship problems
	▶ uncertainty about the decision to be sterilised
	▶ psychiatric illness

Side-effects

There are no effects on the male sexual organs or the male hormones. Sexual libido and functioning should not be affected. Sexual activity can be resumed as soon as a man feels comfortable. Short-term effects include bruising and swelling, which may last for a couple of weeks. This can be minimised by wearing tight underpants for a week, day and night. Heavy lifting work or vigorous sport should be avoided for at least a week.

Scrotal haematoma with or without infection occurs in about six per cent of men who have had a vasectomy, but this is easily treated with antibiotic therapy. It seldom requires more than analgesia and local support, but occasionally can require further treatment.

Sperm granuloma (leakage of sperm into the tissue between the cut ends of the vasa deferentia) causes a foreign body reaction and the formation of discrete tender nodules in about 30 per cent of men with vasectomies. These may cause no problems or they can cause inflammation and pain, which may require treatment by excision of the granuloma.

Sperm antibodies occur in about 60-80 per cent of vasectomised men. (Sperm antibodies are also found less frequently in non-vasectomised men.) As sperm continue to be produced after vasectomy, they are absorbed by the body and testicular antigens can then stimulate an auto-immune response. There is no evidence that sperm antibodies impair immunity or cause any health problems. However, they may reduce the chances of pregnancy after reversal of vasectomy.

Cardiovascular disease, cancer and vasectomy

Worldwide about 42 million couples rely on vasectomy as their method of family planning.

Contrary to earlier reports suggesting a possibility of increased risk of cardiovascular disease, testicular or prostate cancer in men after vasectomy, research to date shows this is not the case.

Ongoing research confirms that men who have had a vasectomy are not at greater risk of any chronic illness or cancer than men who have not undergone the procedure.

As with female sterilisation, psychological problems and regret are uncommon when the decision is well thought out, and where full information and counselling have been available.

Reversibility of male and female sterilisation

Sterilisation is intended to be permanent. However, sometimes reversal is requested because of genuine regret or because of the death of a partner or child, or because there has been a change of relationship. A number of factors influence the success or failure of sterilisation reversal: the method used, for example clips in female sterilisation offer a better potential for reversal than methods that cut or seal the tubes; age of the man or the woman requesting the reversal; and the length of time between the operation and request for reversal (in male sterilisation). The pregnancy rate after vasectomy reversal by expert surgeons can be as high as 90 per cent, but it averages between 20 and 70 per cent. The success rate for female sterilisation reversal depends on the method and the woman's age at reversal. It does not relate to the time interval since the procedure. Where a female sterilisation has been reversed about three to five per cent of pregnancies are ectopic. This compares to 1.5 per cent of all pregnancies being ectopic.

Future methods   New methods are being explored to find easier and more effective ways of blocking the fallopian tubes and vasa deferentia in women and men. These include the use of laser technology, silicone plugs, various chemical agents and new forms of clips.

UK guidelines   In recognition of the diversity in practice in the UK, the RCOG has produced new national guidelines on sterilisation to improve and standardise sterilisation practice, training, information and counselling procedures.

Further reading

Books

Handbook of family planning and reproductive health care
Loudon N, Glasier A and Gebbie A (eds)
3rd edn, Churchill Livingstone, 1995
Chapter 8: Sterilisation, Glasier A

No-scalpel vasectomy – an illustrated guide for surgeons
Gonzales B, Marston-Ainley S and Vansintejan G
Association for Voluntary Surgical Contraception, 1992

Articles

'Fatherhood without apparent spermatozoa after vasectomy'
Smith J C, Cranston D and O'Brien T, et al
The Lancet, 345, 1994, 30

'Classification of azoospermic samples'
Lindsay K, Floyd I and Swan R
The Lancet, 345, 1995, 1642

'The risk of pregnancy after tubal sterilisation: findings from the US Collaborative Review of Sterilisation'
Peterson P B, Xia Z and Hughes J M, et al
American Journal of Obstetrics and Gynecology, 174, 1996, 1161-1170

'Male and female sterilisation: evidence based guidelines no 5'
Royal College of Obstetricians and Gynaecology, 1999

Postcoital contraception

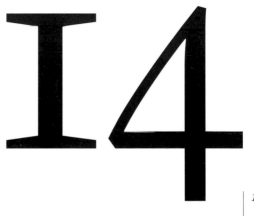

General information

Postcoital or emergency contraception (originally given the misleading name of 'morning after' contraception – this term should not now be used) involves methods that can be given in the event of unprotected intercourse. Unprotected intercourse may be the result of failure to use contraception at all, method failure or problem, default in pill-taking or accidents with a method. Since it is difficult to be sure when some women ovulate in any given cycle, the timing in the cycle for giving this treatment is not precise. Women should always be promptly referred for treatment, even if the risk of pregnancy is small, and in addition this provides the opportunity to discuss future contraception. Postcoital methods should not be used routinely, as postcoital hormonal methods are less effective than regular methods.

General mode of action

Postcoital methods are not abortifacients as they work before implantation and therefore do not disrupt an existing pregnancy. They should not be confused with abortion. It is vitally important that the mode of action is understood in order that accurate information can be given to women considering this method. It should be recognised that for those who believe life begins at fertilisation, as opposed to the medical and legally accepted view that life begins at implantation, these methods may not be acceptable.

If emergency contraception fails, research to date shows no reported fetal abnormalities following the postcoital use of the hormonal methods or the IUD. For this reason, failed emergency contraception is not a medical indication for termination of pregnancy. Outcomes of pregnancy following emergency contraception are routinely collected by the FFPRHC.

The FFPRHC has produced comprehensive guidelines on all methods of emergency contraception.

Hormonal methods

Combined oestrogen/ progestogen methods

Originally, ethinyloestradiol (5mg daily for 5 days) was used effectively for a number of years. Today lower doses of oestrogen with a progestogen are used, as this method has fewer side-effects when compared with the use of oestrogens alone. A combined oestrogen/progestogen formulation can be used, ie 100mcg ethinyloestradiol plus 500mcg levonorgestrel (equivalent to 2 tablets of Ovran) repeated once 12 hours later. This is known as the Yuzpe method. Schering PC4 is marketed specifically as a postcoital contraceptive. Although Ovran is not licensed for emergency contraception, a medical practitioner can prescribe it for this purpose provided full responsibility for this is taken and suitable verbal and written information is given to the client.

In June 1996, the Reproductive Health Drugs Advisory Committee of the US Food and Drug Administration (FDA) confirmed the safety and effectiveness of methods of certain oral contraceptives as emergency contraceptive pills.

If emergency hormonal contraception is required by a client using liver enzyme inducing drugs such as rifampicin, it is suggested that 3 tablets are taken, with another 3 tablets 12 hours later (total dose – 6 tablets). Current (1999) pharmacological opinion suggests there is no need to increase the dose for women using antibiotics.

Mode of action

This is considered to be multifactorial and mainly includes:

▶ rendering the endometrium unfavourable for implantation
▶ desynchronisation of the delicate sequential effects relating to ovum transport
▶ prevention or delay in ovulation if given early enough in the cycle
▶ alteration of normal corpus luteum function which results in a shortened luteal phase

Efficacy

Effectiveness rates vary between 95 and 99 per cent. The overall risk of pregnancy after a single act of unprotected intercourse on any day of the menstrual cycle is 2-4 per cent. The pregnancy risk from a single act of intercourse is highest near to and at ovulation, being between 20-30 per cent. 1998 WHO research shows that combined hormonal emergency contraception is most effective when used within 24 hours of sex.

Timing and use of hormonal methods

Hormonal methods can be given up to 72 hours (3 days) of unprotected intercourse. Treatment should be initiated as soon as it is practicable after the episode of unprotected intercourse as efficacy is improved. Women who contact services should not have appointments delayed to the next day even if this still falls within the 72 hour limit. Continued contraception should be advised during this time. There is no age limit, even in smokers. Treatment can be repeated in a menstrual cycle if required. It is important where possible to take the first dose at a time which will enable the second dose to be taken at a convenient time 12 hours later.

Contra-indications

▶ pregnancy/suspected pregnancy
▶ migraine at presentation in a woman with focal migraine history
▶ breast-feeding – relative contraindication if feeding is not established (which it should be by the time a woman would be at possible risk – three weeks after childbirth). If a woman feels uneasy about having a hormonal method while breast-feeding, she can express her breast milk during this time
▶ past history of thrombosis – relative contraindication

Side-effects

The main side-effects are nausea and vomiting. Nausea may occur in up to 50 per cent of cases. Vomiting may occur in up to 24 per cent. An anti-emetic such as Motilium (domperidone) can be prescribed to reduce the occurrence and severity of nausea. Nausea and vomiting may be reduced if food is taken with the tablets. In addition, some women experience headaches, dizziness or breast tenderness. If vomiting occurs within 2 hours of taking either set of pills, the dose should be repeated or the possibility of an IUD insertion should be discussed.

Women should be advised that following hormonal postcoital contraception, the next period may be earlier or later than usual or on time. A few women have light bleeding shortly after taking hormonal postcoital contraception. This should not be confused with a period.

Progestogen-only methods

Several progestogen-only emergency contraception (POEC) formulations have been used. The Ho and Kwan method utilised 2 doses, each of 0.75mg levonorgestrel (equivalent to 25 tablets of Microval or Norgeston or 20 tablets of Neogest) taken 12 hours apart and initiated within 48 hours of intercourse. Efficacy was equivalent to the Yuzpe method.

New research by WHO (1998) confirms and extends that of Ho and Kwan. The research provides evidence that:

▶ levonorgestrel (0.75mg repeated after 12 hours) is significantly more effective in preventing pregnancy than the Yuzpe method when given up to 72 hours after unprotected sexual intercourse - 1.1 per cent failure rate
▶ efficacy is improved if given within 24 hours after unprotected sexual intercourse - 0.4 per cent failure rate
▶ side-effects of nausea and vomiting are much reduced with POEC methods

There are few absolute contradictions to POEC methods, only current or suspected pregnancy. Specific licensed products are expected to be available in 1999.

Intrauterine contraceptive devices

IUDs can be inserted as a postcoital method. The levonorgestrel IUS is not recommended for postcoital use as it is not effective.

Mode of action

The presence of an IUD will prevent implantation by inducing changes in the endometrium. The copper also affects the biochemical process and enzymes involved in implantation. Data on the emergency use of an IUD confirm that it does not act as an abortifacient as implantation and subsequent pregnancy does not occur before 5-7 days after fertilisation.

Efficacy

IUDs used postcoitally are almost 100 per cent effective. Only four documented failures have been reported.

When efficacy is a priority the IUD is the emergency contraceptive method of choice. It can also be used as an ongoing long-term method, where appropriate. In the very rare case of an IUD failing, and the woman wishes to continue with the pregnancy, the device should be removed if accessible (see 'IUDs', page 104). If the device is not to be left in place, then it is removed towards the end of the next menstrual period.

Timing of use of IUDs postcoitally

The IUD is effective up to 5 days after unprotected sexual intercourse and can also be fitted in good faith up to 5 days after the earliest calculation of ovulation.

Contra-indications

▶ suspected pregnancy
▶ past history of ectopic pregnancy (relative contraindication if IUD is removed at next period)
▶ special care is needed in cases of sexual assault or unsure STI/PID histories – STI screening and/or antibiotic cover should be considered

Side-effects

These are the same as for IUDs in general (see page 100). The possibility of an STI should always be checked.

General

All present methods of postcoital contraception are effective and safe. It is essential that full information and counselling take place before postcoital contraception is used, and appropriate follow-up arranged.

Postcoital contraception is easily available from most general practitioners, community family planning clinics and many genitourinary clinics (hormonal rather than IUDs).

The risks of postcoital contraception are small and are outweighed by the benefits of preventing an unwanted pregnancy.

A 1994 consensus meeting on the provision of emergency contraception held at the RCOG of all the family planning organisations and the RCOG, the RCGP, the Health Education Authority, The Royal Pharmaceutical Society of Great Britain (RPSGB) and the RCN, looked at widening the availability of postcoital contraception to include provision through nurses and pharmacists. There was unanimous agreement for the need to widen availability in order to improve awareness and uptake.

Follow-up

All women receiving postcoital contraception should be offered the opportunity to attend for follow-up within three to four weeks or earlier if a period is missed or if she is concerned or worried. This can provide a further opportunity to talk about future contraception, and any other sexual health or contraceptive issues.

Future methods

Anti-progestogens have been researched for use as emergency contraceptives. Research by WHO on the use of mifepristone as a postcoital method has been found to be highly successful using a single dose of 600mg. Fewer side-effects occurred than with the Yuzpe method. The minimum effective dose and time period in which it can be used effectively still have to be defined.

Other hormones are being researched as postcoital methods, including different progestogens.

Further reading

Book

The provision of emergency hormonal contraception
Paintin D (ed)
RCOG Press, 1995

Resources

Recommendations for clinical practice: Emergency contraception
Faculty of Family Planning and Reproductive Health Care of the RCOG, 1998

Emergency contraception audit kit
National Co-ordinating Unit for Clinical Audit in Family Planning, 1995
available from the FFPRHC

Articles

'Randomised controlled trial of levonorgestrel versus the Yuzpe regimen of combined oral contraceptives for emergency contraception'
Task Force on Postovulatory Methods of Fertility Regulations, WHO
The Lancet, 352, 1998, 428-433

'Time for emergency contraception with levonorgestrel alone'
Guillebaud J
The Lancet, 352, 1998, 416-417
The Lancet, 352, 1998, 658 (correction)

Contraceptive developments

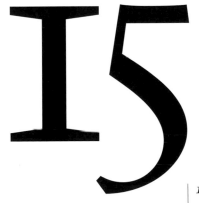

General information

The idea of a new method of contraception, perhaps as big a breakthrough as the pill was in the early 1960s, always fascinates the popular press. Reports that male pills, contraceptive nasal sprays, vaccines, and once a month methods are 'just around the corner' have appeared repeatedly in newspapers and women's magazines, and on television during the last 25 years. As a result, health professionals may be asked about such new methods and whether they are generally available yet. Unfortunately the answer is 'no'. Despite the hope that such methods will ultimately become available, they are at least five to 10 years away. The time it takes for transition of a new idea to a final product can be up to 20 years or longer. Unfortunately, issues relating to funding, increasing litigation and limited availability may mean that future choice of method may be limited rather than enhanced.

Table 12 Summary of contraceptive developments

Hormonal – 'variations on a theme'

Oral contraceptives	► newer refined pills offering lower doses and 'safer' hormones
Injectables	► refinements in dosage ► different progestogens such as levonorgestrel butanoate ► combined hormones ► different time periods – monthly, 3 monthly, annual
Implants	► long-acting rod systems ► biodegradable systems of progestogen ► combinations of oestrogen and progestogen
Vaginal rings	► vaginal delivery of oestrogen and/or progestogen ► use of natural progesterone
Hormonal patches/gels	► transdermal hormone delivery
Intracervical devices	► devices placed between the uterus and vagina delivering hormones
Male pill	► hormone pills ► hormone injections
GnRH agonists	► nasal sprays or other antagonist of GnRH

Intrauterine devices

Modified IUDs	► flexible and frameless IUDs ► different or modified shapes ► longer-lasting IUDs

Barrier methods

Diaphragms and caps ▶ modified designs
▶ different materials substituting synthetic materials for latex

Male and female condoms

▶ modified designs
▶ different materials substituting synthetic materials for latex

Spermicides

▶ newer compounds offering improved spermicidal, microbiocidal and virucidal activity

Natural family planning/fertility awareness

▶ improvement in the range and choice of effective fertility devices/systems to help identify the fertile and infertile times of the menstrual cycle (measuring changes in urine, vaginal secretions, cervical mucus, saliva)
▶ more research and understanding and improved usage of lactational amenorrhoea

Sterilisation

▶ agents to block the tubes such as silicone plugs
▶ research into 'reversible' methods
▶ new clips for blocking the vasa deferentia (vasoclude clips)

Vaccines

▶ research into immunological methods to prevent pregnancy:
anti-hCG vaccines
anti-sperm and ova vaccines
anti-zona pellucida vaccines

Postcoital contraception

▶ anti-progestogens
▶ different hormones

Further reading

Books

Developing new contraceptives – obstacles and opportunities
Mastrianni L, Donaldson P J and Kate T (eds)
Committee on Contraceptive Development
National Academy Press, 1990
John Wiley and Sons Ltd (distributor, UK)

UNDP/UNFPA/WHO
World Bank Special Programme of Research, Development and Research Training in Human Reproduction – Reproductive Health Research: the new directions – Biennial Report 1996-7
WHO, Geneva, 1998

Pregnancy testing

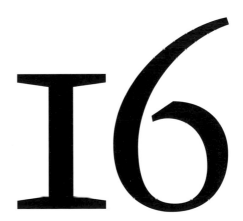

General information

Early identification of pregnancy enables early up-take of ante-natal care and improved healthcare for pregnancy, when the pregnancy is wanted. It facilitates the early diagnosis of any pregnancy problem, multiple pregnancy or fetal abnormality. In addition, and importantly, it provides time for a woman (and her partner) to make choices in the event of an unplanned pregnancy.

Pregnancy tests are carried out in a variety of places: hospitals, outpatient clinics, community family planning clinics, in general practice, young people's clinics or centres, pregnancy advisory centres and some GUM clinics. However, because of limited resources within the NHS and changes in services offered by primary care professionals, pregnancy testing is becoming more difficult to obtain quickly and easily on the NHS. Many pharmacies now offer a pregnancy testing service and sell 'home pregnancy testing kits'.

Pregnancy testing should be readily available in general practice and in community family planning clinics. Some GPs and clinics send pregnancy tests to local laboratories, which may mean waiting longer for the result. Results are usually available within a minimum of two days, but some laboratories take considerably longer. Where pregnancy testing is undertaken in general practice, the results are immediate. Privacy, appropriate information and counselling should always be available and the results should be given with due sensitivity: a pregnancy may be very much wanted or not wanted at all. Time may be needed to 'take-in' the result of a test, and there may be a need to return at a later time for discussion.

Pregnancy testing in pharmacies

Pregnancy testing is a professional service offered by many community pharmacists. Any service should be offered with sensitivity and care. The following guidelines have been issued by the Council of the Royal Pharmaceutical Society which operates a strict code of practice:

Confidentiality

The pharmacist must keep all information provided by the patient and the result of the test confidential and only disclose information with the consent of the patient. Advice on contraception may be sought at the same time as a pregnancy test and the pharmacist is reminded of the guidance notes contained in the code of ethics on contraceptive advice to girls under 16.

Advertising

Pregnancy testing is regarded as a professional service and therefore should only be advertised in accordance with the relevant parts of Principle 7 of the Code of Ethics.

Facilities for carrying out the test

A reliable method of testing should be used. In order to prevent contamination which can be caused by handling samples of urine, the testing should take place in a separate room from the one used for dispensing. The room should be kept clean and tidy and all working surfaces should be finished with a smooth, impervious and washable material. Adequate lighting should be provided so that the results of the test can be read correctly. A separate sink should be provided.

Procedures which ensure that no confusion occurs between samples must be devised and followed.

People carrying out tests should wash their hands before leaving the working area.

All cuts and grazes on hands or exposed parts of the body must be covered with waterproof dressings.

Request for a pregnancy test

A signed and dated confirmation of the request should be obtained. The form on which confirmation is obtained should state the limits of accuracy of the test. All questions relating to the test should be asked by the pharmacist and the answers recorded in writing.

Records

A written record of the result of the test, together with information provided by the patient and the type of test and batch number of the test materials, should be retained by the pharmacist for at least one year. Such records must be stored safely to preserve confidentiality.

Communication of the result

The result of the test should be provided in writing on a standard form. If it is necessary to give the result by telephone, the pharmacist should be satisfied that the person requesting the information is the person who requested the test.

A written confirmation of the result should be provided even when the result has been communicated by telephone.

The form should be dated and give the name and address of the patient. The result should be given as positive or negative with an explanation of such terms and the limits of accuracy of the test, eg 'The specimen provided has been tested for urinary gonadotrophin and has been found to be positive/negative. Research has shown the results of the test to be accurate in 98 per cent of all cases. A positive result indicates a probable pregnancy'. At the request of the client a copy of the form should be sent to her medical practitioner. Notwithstanding the result of the test, the patient should be strongly advised to consult her medical practitioner or, if she appears reluctant to do so, another source of medical advice, eg a pregnancy advisory bureau. The pharmacist should not recommend a particular pregnancy advisory bureau but should have a list available for use if the patient requests information.

Advice from the pharmacist

The pharmacist can clearly provide invaluable support in this area, especially if a woman is undecided or ambivalent about the pregnancy. Pharmacists can provide appropriate information to refer the woman immediately for further information, counselling and medical help.

Many pharmacists now have quieter, more discreet areas where discussion can be relatively private.

Home pregnancy tests

The vast majority of pharmacies sell 'do-it-yourself pregnancy testing kits' such as Clear Blue, Predictor and Discover Today. Modern pregnancy tests are about 98 per cent accurate if the instructions are carried out correctly, and can be used from the first day the period is missed.

False results

False negative results

Home pregnancy tests are not difficult to carry out. However, there may be problems in following the instructions, especially if a woman is nervous about the outcome of the test. False negative results are not common and if they do occur they are much more likely than false positives with all kinds of pregnancy tests. False negative results can be due to:

▶ too little, too dilute, or too old urine
▶ traces of detergent in the urine container
▶ carrying out the test too soon (before a missed period)
▶ disturbing the test (not an issue with dip stick tests)

A false negative result can also be due to medical causes, such as ectopic pregnancy or a miscarriage. Because of this a false negative result in the absence of a period should be investigated further.

False positive results

False positive results can be due to:

▶ raised hCG for reasons other than pregnancy
▶ raised gonadotrophins around the menopause
▶ heavy proteinuria or haematuria
▶ drugs such as fertility drugs

Problems in early pregnancy

Now that pregnancy can be confirmed so early, there is a greater awareness of miscarriage, and the fact that many pregnancies do not go to term. About 15-20 per cent of pregnancies are lost in the first three months. Any woman who has any bleeding and/or lower abdominal pain early in pregnancy should be investigated without delay. Such a pregnancy may continue, be miscarried or be ectopic. Ectopic pregnancy occurs in 1.5 per cent of all pregnancies, and accounts for up to 10 per cent of maternal mortality.

Abortion

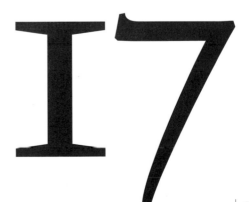

Abortion is not considered to be a method of contraception. However it is an important and necessary back-up to family planning services, especially as no method of contraception is 100 per cent effective. As such it *should* be part of the range of sexual health services.

The Abortion Act 1967

Before 1967 abortion was legal only to save the life of the mother. The 1967 Abortion Act extended the grounds for legal abortion in England, Wales and Scotland. It does not apply to Northern Ireland.

Under the Act, legal termination of pregnancy may be carried out provided that two registered medical practitioners agree that it is necessary on one or more of the following grounds:

▶ the continuance of the pregnancy would involve risk to the life of the pregnant woman, or of injury to her physical or mental health, or that of any existing children, greater than if the pregnancy were terminated
▶ there is substantial risk of the child being born handicapped

In determining the risk of injury to health of the woman or her children, the woman's actual or reasonably foreseeable future environment may be taken into account. No person is obliged to perform or participate in an abortion to which they have a conscientious objection. A doctor who conscientiously objects to abortion should quickly refer a woman to a colleague who does not have such objections. If the pregnant woman is married, her husband's consent is not required. Where a young woman is under 16, it is not absolutely essential to obtain parental consent to have an abortion. However, it is usually in a young person's interest for her to inform and involve her parents/guardians. Where there is refusal to do so, it is important to find out if she will involve another adult whom she feels she can trust. Where this proves to be impossible, most hospitals have social welfare support, and can establish that she understands the consequences of her decision and is capable of giving consent. Alternatively, young people's clinics such as Brook have counsellors skilled in this area.

In the UK, the Children Act 1989 established the right for young people to give consent to their own medical treatment, which includes contraception and abortion, regardless of their age, providing they are capable of giving consent and understanding the issues.

Very few abortions are carried out in women under 16 without parental involvement. Often with good support and trust young people can be enabled to talk with their parents either alone or with another sympathetic person present.

Abortion services are controlled by Department of Health regulations. This includes the medical methods of abortion (mifepristone use). Except in an emergency, abortion may take place only in an NHS hospital or in a private nursing home approved for this purpose by the Department of Health. Most non-NHS abortions take place in charitable clinics run by the British Pregnancy Advisory Service (BPAS) or the Marie Stopes Clinic, both of which have clinics in cities throughout the country.

1990 amendment to the 1967 Abortion Act

The Abortion Act 1967 was amended by Section 37 of the Human Fertilisation and Embryology Act which became law in 1991. The amendment does not modify the general principles of the original act, and does not alter the basis of access to abortion. The amendment covers three areas:

It introduced a new upper time limit of 24 weeks for legal abortion, although no upper time limit applies in a few extreme specified circumstances. These are:

- ▶ risk to the life of the mother
- ▶ risk of grave permanent injury to the mother
- ▶ risk of serious fetal handicap

It included selective induced abortion in a multiple pregnancy under the terms of the Abortion Act 1967.

It authorised the Secretary of State for Health to approve a new class of places for the purposes of medical termination of pregnancy. This prepared the way for the licensing of places appropriate to medical methods of abortion using drugs.

Because the 1967 Abortion Act does not extend to Northern Ireland, abortion is not available except in exceptional circumstances, such as to save the mother's life. Those who choose the option of abortion in Northern Ireland may travel to Britain to obtain an abortion privately. (Women from Northern Ireland are not eligible for NHS treatment.)

Public opinion and views

The extent to which legislation follows or influences public opinion is debatable. Opinion polls show that although abortion continues to be a controversial and diverse issue, attitudes have become more liberal.

The annual British Social Attitudes Survey reveals that in the 1980s attitudes towards the social and medical grounds for abortion became significantly more liberal. These views have not changed in the 1990s. Polls carried out in 1991 (Harris), 1993 (Gallup) and 1995, 1996 (Mori) all indicate a majority view that abortion should be available on request.

Availability

There is no legal requirement for health authorities to provide an abortion service. The level of provision varies considerably between districts from very good to extremely poor.

Charitable abortion clinics within the private sector developed after the 1967 Act was passed, to meet needs which could not be met by the NHS at that time. The continuing importance of private sector abortions largely reflects continuing inadequacies in NHS provision for abortion. Some private services are contracted to provide NHS abortion services.

Private abortion clinics have to be classed as approved places for termination of pregnancy and are closely regulated by the Department of Health.

Counselling and information

Pregnancy counselling and information should always be available for women who have an unplanned pregnancy. Informed, non-directive counselling allows a woman (and her partner) to be sure of any decision made with regard to continuing or terminating a pregnancy.

Methods of abortion

Surgical techniques

In practice, most abortions are carried out within the first 12 weeks of pregnancy (first trimester). Up to this time abortions can be carried out safely by techniques such as vacuum aspiration or dilatation and curettage (D&C).

Vacuum aspiration
In vacuum aspiration, the cervix is dilated and the womb is emptied by suction through a thin plastic tube. The procedure is usually carried out under a light general anaesthetic or less usually under local anaesthetic.

Dilatation and curettage (D&C)
In a D&C, the cervix is dilated first and a curette is introduced into the womb to remove the contents. It is carried out under general anaesthetic.

Abortions carried out after 12 weeks (second trimester abortions) can be more difficult, with a higher complication rate. There are two methods:

Dilatation and evacuation (D&E)
In a D&E, the cervix is dilated first and the contents of the womb – fetus and placenta – are removed with special forceps. The uterus is further emptied by vacuum

aspiration. It is carried out under general anaesthetic. This method can be used up to 20 weeks, but most hospitals prefer to use medical induction after 16 weeks.

Medical induction
Medical induction involves inducing labour: usually prostaglandin is administered by vaginal pessary or intravenous infusion (IVI) injections. Drugs used to stimulate labour at full term can also be used. The fetus is expelled. Late abortions are carried out infrequently.

Medical methods

Anti-progestogens
Anti-progestogens work by blocking the action of progesterone which is necessary for the maintenance of the pregnancy.

The use of mifepristone marketed as Mifegyne, provides a medical alternative for some women to the presently available surgical techniques of abortion. This method can be used in the first nine weeks of pregnancy (63 days from the first day of the last period) and involves the use of mifepristone, with a prostaglandin. It is highly effective. Medical abortion using mifepristone is not suitable for smokers over the age of 35. Since 1995 mifepristone has also been licensed for the medical induction of termination of pregnancy between 13 and 20 weeks gestation.

Further reading

Books
Modern methods of inducing abortion
Baird DT, Grimes DA and Van Look P (eds)
Blackwell Science, 1995

Unplanned pregnancy – your choices
Furedi A
Oxford University Press, 1996

Unplanned pregnancy – making the right choices for you
Klein D and Kaufmann T
Thorsons, 1996

Legal and ethical issues

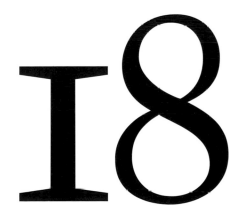

**General
information**

The Family Law Reform Act 1969 (Section 8) in England provides that the consent to medical or surgical treatment of an individual who has attained the age of 16 shall be effective consent, and that in such cases it is not necessary to obtain consent from a parent or guardian. The medical age of consent is also 16 in Scotland and in Northern Ireland. In general, family planning services, methods and supplies are available to all, irrespective of age, sex or marital status.

**Confidentiality
and medical
consultation**

The confidential nature of the patient-doctor relationship is of historic and fundamental importance to communication between individuals and care/counselling professionals. For people over the age of 16, the right of confidentiality is absolute, except under particular circumstances defined by the General Medical Council. Adult individuals have the right to expect that personal information, directly or indirectly given, will not be gratuitously disclosed or used to their detriment and that no third party, unless directly involved in their care, will have legitimate access to information about their medical condition or personal circumstances.

Under-16s

For people under the age of 16, the situation is less clear. Many young people are unsure whether or not they can expect confidentiality and many doctors are unaware that they are legally able to offer confidential consultation and treatment.

The provision of written or verbal information, services or prescription of family planning methods to under-16s is legal without parental consent throughout the United Kingdom. Public attention in England was drawn to the dilemmas concerning contraception and the under-16s by the 'Gillick' case.

The decision whether or not to prescribe contraception for a person under 16 without parental consent ultimately rests with the clinical judgment of the doctor.

Specific advice and guidance are provided to doctors, health authorities and other health professionals by the Department of Health in its 1986 circular, *Family planning services for young people.* (This replaced Section G of the *Family planning service memorandum of guidance 1974.*) This circular relates only to England and Wales. The equivalent Scottish circular, the *National health circular 1974,* makes no mention of the under-16s, but provides advice that services should be available to all. Under the Age of Legal Capacity (Scotland) Act 1991, under-16s may consent to medical treatment if, in the opinion of the doctor, they are capable of understanding the nature and consequences of any proposed treatment. In Northern Ireland the situation regarding the under-16s is the same as that applying in England.

The Department of Health's guidance to doctors and health professionals includes several areas of advice. In considering the provision of advice or treatment on contraception doctors and other professional staff need to take special care not to undermine parental responsibility and family stability. The doctor or other professional should therefore always seek to persuade the young person to tell the parents or guardian (or other person in loco parentis), or to let him or her inform them that advice or treatment is given.

There will be cases where it is not possible to persuade the young person either to inform the parents or to allow the doctor or other professional to do so. This may be, for example, where family relationships have broken down. In such cases, a doctor or other professional would be justified in giving advice and treatment without parental knowledge or consent, provided they were satisfied:

▶ that the young person could understand the advice and had sufficient maturity to understand what was involved in terms of the moral, social and emotional implications

▶ that they could neither persuade the young person to inform the parents, nor to allow him/her to inform them, that contraceptive advice was being sought

▶ that the young person would be very likely to begin, or to continue having, sexual intercourse with or without contraceptive treatment

▶ that, without contraceptive advice or treatment, the young person's physical or mental health, or both, would be likely to suffer

▶ that the young person's best interests required them to give contraceptive advice, treatment or both without parental consent

The Children Act 1989 strongly supports the notion of young people's rights, and emphasises the responsibilities (rather than rights) of parents. Department of Health guidelines relating to this legislation state that 'children under 16 may also be able to give or refuse consent depending upon their capacity to understand the nature of the treatment, it is for the doctor to decide this'.

A guidance document was issued jointly in 1993 by the BMA, GMSC, Brook Advisory Centres, **fpa**, HEA and RCGP. This document, issued as clarification of good medical practice, identifies two key General Medical Council rulings, namely that:

Any competent young person, regardless of age, can independently seek medical advice and give valid consent to medical treatment. Competency is understood in terms of the young person's ability to understand the choices available and their consequences, including any risk factors. While it may be preferable, parental consent to treatment is not necessary.

The duty of confidentiality owed to a person under 16 is as great as the duty owed to any other person. Confidentiality should be respected concerning the consultation, whether or not treatment is provided, unless there are very convincing reasons to the contrary;

doctors must be prepared to justify any decisions to breach confidentiality before the General Medical Council.

Confidentiality and school nurses and teachers

Confidentiality of medical consultation is covered by the ethical principles of the profession. Others involved in the care of people under the age of 16 work with less clear guidance.

School nursing provision varies enormously, with some schools having a full-time school nurse, others having limited access. At the time of writing school nursing arrangements are under review by most health trusts in England. School nursing today can involve a number of different responsibilities which include health promotion, education and counselling in addition to health screening. As such the school nurse (and other health professionals) now play an important role in the area of school sex education.

In order that the school nurse's position is clear in relation to working with young people under 16 there is a need to understand the difference between a health professional giving medical advice about contraception, and a teacher or health professional giving general information about contraception in a classroom setting. School nurses are subject to the UKCC Code of Professional Conduct when working on an individual basis with a pupil. Confidential medical advice can be given to individual pupils about contraception, providing they follow the Department of Health guidelines.

When a school nurse is contributing to the school sex education programme in a classroom setting, the nurse is working as part of the education team and must work within the sex education policy of the school. It is good practice for the different roles of the school nurse to be clarified in school settings.

Confidentiality of records

The Data Protection Act 1984, which relates to computerised records, and Access to Health Records Act 1990 gave all people the right to access their records from that date. Where a person under 16 applies for access to their records they must be able to demonstrate that they are capable of understanding the nature of the application. A parent or guardian of a young person below the age of 16 will not be given access to records unless the young person has given their consent or is incapable of understanding the nature of the application, and the granting of access would be in their best interests.

Further reading

Book
Sex and the law: a brief guide for staff working with people with learning difficulties
4th edition
Gunn MJ
fpa, 1996

Booklets
Confidentiality and people under 16
Guidance issued jointly by the BMA, GMSC, Brook Advisory Centres, **fpa**, HEA and RCGP
BMA, 1993

What should I do?
Guidance on confidentiality and under 16s for community nurses, social workers, teachers and youth workers
Brook Advisory Centres, 1996

'Someone with a smile would be your best bet – what young people want from sex advice services'
Brook Advisory Centres, 1998

Reproductive health and sexual health services

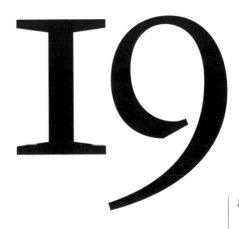

General information

All addresses of organisations listed in this chapter can be found under 'Addresses of useful organisations' on pages 198-209.

Contraception is an important part of reproductive health, but there are also many other health issues that may be raised or addressed during a contraceptive consultation. People may well raise related issues such as planning for a family or having a healthy pregnancy, difficulties in conceiving, concern about sexually transmitted infections, the menopause etc. It is helpful if professionals can provide information and addresses of services or help organisations and refer the person to an appropriate source of help.

Young people's services

Nearly all health authorities have young people's services. Details of individual services can be obtained from the **fpa**'s Contraceptive Education Service. Brook Advisory Centres welcome under-25s. Young people's services provide much more than just contraceptive services; information, counselling, help and support are provided on all personal and relationship problems. Youth Access is an organisation that provides full details about young people's counselling services.

Brook Advisory Centres

These are family planning clinics providing special services for young people (up to 25) which were set up in 1964. They help with any contraception advice and supplies, help with any sexual, emotional or relationship problems and provide pregnancy testing and pregnancy counselling. Most services are free, but a fee is payable at some clinics. There are clinics throughout the UK. Brook also produces leaflets, booklets, education resources and other literature.

Sexually transmitted infections including HIV

Any person concerned or worried about a possible STI, including HIV, should receive help and advice or be referred to a genitourinary medicine (GUM) clinic. In the UK, the Venereal Disease Regulations (1916) allowed for the establishment of clinics for the diagnosis and treatment in confidence of sexually transmitted infections. In addition to diagnosis and treatment, trained counsellors and health advisers are available to provide information, help and support and some GUM/sexual health clinics provide psychosexual services. GUM clinics can be found attached to most large hospitals.

Contraception and sexually transmitted infections

Contraceptive methods, in addition to preventing unplanned pregnancy, can in some cases protect against STIs. Until recently, contraceptive technology development, policy emphasis and service delivery have focused mainly on preventing pregnancy, with little attention being paid to prevention of STIs. In the UK, services for providing contraception are entirely separate from those services for diagnosis and treatment of STIs – they are financed from different budgets, often situated in separate buildings and run by staff with a different approach, training and career structure. However, more recently the need for collaboration has been recognised with an increasing number of GUM clinics now providing contraceptive services with trained family planning staff. Studies show that many women attending GUM clinics require contraceptive advice and those attending family planning clinics need advice on STIs. Many areas of the country are now developing sexual health services recognising the need for holistic sexual health and reproductive health services for women and men.

There are a number of organisations and groups set up to help people concerned or worried about HIV and AIDS (see page 207).

Sexual problems

Professionals working in the area of sexual and reproductive health may become involved in addressing sexual problems. GPs, nurses and other members of the health team may become involved because sexual problems affect overall health. Sexual history-taking is now a recommended practice and this can provide an opportunity for a person to raise issues and seek advice.

Not all health professionals, however, feel competent or comfortable about discussing sexual matters. Good listening and understanding are important and providing simple advice is often all that might be required. Where this is not the case, specialist psychosexual help should be considered. Psychosexual counselling is available through some community family planning clinics and a number of GPs and doctors are now trained in psychosexual medicine. RELATE also provides help with sexual difficulties through trained sex therapists.

The Institute of Psychosexual Medicine can also help with enquiries about practitioners trained in psychosexual medicine and can provide information about training.

Relationship/ marriage problems

Counselling and help may be obtained from:

- ▶ RELATE
- ▶ London Marriage Guidance Council
- ▶ Marriage Care
- ▶ Marriage Counselling Scotland
- ▶ Jewish Marriage Council

Well-woman services

Well-woman services provide screening for breast and cervical cancer, instruction in breast self-examination and awareness, blood pressure checks etc, in symptom-free women.

Those seeking well-woman services without contraceptive advice can go to a well-woman clinic without referral by a GP. These clinics are run by some health authorities as part of the community services. Some private clinics also exist.

Well-man services

Well-man services exist in a few areas and provide sexual health services and, sometimes, general health screening in general practice and community clinics.

Cervical smears and breast awareness

Cervical smears are carried out by GPs or practice nurses in general practice, or as part of a contraceptive service at family planning clinics. Every woman who has ever had heterosexual sex should be invited to have a cervical smear every three to five years between the ages of 20-64. Screening for cervical cancer has been in place in the UK since 1967. In the late 1980s the National Co-ordinating Network (NCN) was set up to provide an effective screening programme. In 1994 a National Co-ordinator was appointed to administer both cervical and breast screening programmes for the UK. The NCN publishes a wide range of literature for professionals covering guidelines, training, audit, clinical practice and management, etc. Breast checks are also carried out at family planning clinics and as necessary by primary health care professionals. Breast cancer screening using mammography is nationally available for women between the ages of 50-64. Women over 50 are invited to have routine breast screening (mammography) every three years. Women should be encouraged to be aware of their breasts and therefore aware of any changes. Leaflets are available from the Women's Nationwide Cancer Control Campaign (WNCCC), CancerBACUP and the HEA.

Pre-pregnancy care

Pre-pregnancy care can help women and their partners to prepare for pregnancy both physically and emotionally. It also provides an opportunity for health professionals to discuss relevant issues, such as any potentially inherited disorders. Genetic counselling is available within each region and people can self-refer. Other aspects, such as nutrition, diet, folic acid, rubella, exercise, smoking, health and work should also be discussed.

Infertility

About 10-15 per cent of couples are infertile, this being defined as pregnancy not occurring after one year of trying for a baby. Considerable unhappiness may be experienced by a couple who find themselves infertile. There is often a feeling of isolation among those who have a fertility problem, as they may feel that no one else can understand their situation.

Two main organisations are available to help with infertility in the UK:

- ► ISSUE
- ► CHILD

There are also a number of hospital fertility units which provide support groups. The Human Fertilisation and Embryology Authority (HFEA) provides lists of clinics offering help as well as having a national regulatory role.

Premenstrual syndrome

The premenstrual syndrome (PMS) is characterised by a group of symptoms which may occur in the second half of a woman's menstrual cycle just before her period. These symptoms, which vary from woman to woman, include depression, irritability, headaches, fluid retention and tiredness. Today there is a better understanding of PMS and this has led to improved forms of help and treatment.

Women should be encouraged to seek help from their GP. Some family planning clinics provide help. There are a few NHS specialist PMS clinics. Organisations such as PREMSOC and the National Association of PMS (NAPS) can help with advice and support.

Menopause

The menopause or change of life is the time when a woman's periods finally cease. Cyclical changes in hormone output may be disturbed for several months before the menopause, and women may experience symptoms due to oestrogen deficiency for some time after their periods cease. Not all women find the menopause a troublesome time in life; many pass smoothly through it. Others are severely affected by certain symptoms and require help and advice.

Oestrogen replacement in the form of hormone replacement therapy (HRT) is available in a variety of different preparations depending on specific need. The recognised benefits of oestrogen replacement (eg prevention of osteoporosis) need to be weighed up against possible disadvantages (eg issues around possible increased risk of breast cancer).

Menopausal symptoms include hot flushes or cold sweats, numbness and tingling, vaginal dryness, nervousness and irritability, depression and poor sleep.

Women seeking help should be referred to their own doctor in the first instance or to a menopause clinic. The Amarant Centre and the National Osteoporosis Society can provide help and advice. The British Menopause Society provides advice for professionals.

Contraception and the menopause

The recommended medical guidelines from the Medical Advisory Committees of the **fpa** and the FPPRHC are that contraceptive methods should be continued until a woman has not had a period or any bleeding for two years if she is aged under 50, or one year if she is over 50.

*The **fpa**'s Contraceptive Education Service and Helpline can provide full information on all aspects of contraception, reproductive and sexual health, including details of UK service provision (see '**fpa** services', page 213).*

Note

See 'Addresses of useful organisations' on pages 198-209.

Family planning training

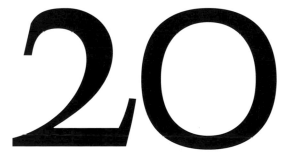

Clinical training

Fertility and reproductive health issues are now a recognised part of undergraduate medical training. The **fpa** is committed to the view that all professionals providing contraceptive services should be trained and have a recognised postgraduate family planning qualification.

The Diploma of the FFPRHC (DFFP) has replaced the UK Joint Committee on Contraception (JCC) certificate in family planning for doctors. Qualification for the Faculty Diploma involves the theoretical and practical training at approved training centres and by Faculty-approved instructing doctors. Additional certification is required for IUD and implant insertion. As innovative methods become available in the future, training, where appropriate, will be established by the Faculty.

Family planning training for nurses is available through the English, Scottish, Northern Ireland and Welsh National Boards of Nursing. The revised framework for post registration education in family planning and reproductive sexual health (FP & RSH) includes: ENB 9903 – Foundation in Family Planning and Reproductive Sexual Health Care, ENB 8103 – The Practice of Family Planning and Reproductive Sexual Health Care and ENB S103 – Clinical Specialist in Family Planning and Reproductive Sexual Health Care Specialist Practitioner Qualification. In addition, some areas may have access to the ENB R71 (revised ENB 901).

Natural family planning (NFP) training is available to medical professionals and non-medical professionals. Accredited training is available from Fertility UK.

Training in psychosexual medicine

The Institute of Psychosexual Medicine offers training to doctors to improve their skills with clients who seek help with sexual difficulties. Doctors attending courses of seminar training may present themselves for the Institute Diploma exam during their 5th term of training.

Further training can lead to eligibility for the membership examination of the Institute.

The Association of Sexual and Marital Therapists provides research, training and skills to medical and health professionals.

The Association of Psychosexual Nursing offers Balint style training seminars for nurses.

Non-clinical training

Family planning is not primarily a medical issue. The role of a family planning service is to empower clients to take responsibility for, and to exercise choice over, their sexual and reproductive health, and to provide support for those experiencing difficulties in relation to their sexuality. While the provision of contraception clearly requires medical knowledge and skills, a comprehensive family planning service is as much about non-medical health education and health promotion, and the provision of advice, information and counselling.

Training about sexuality in all its aspects and in counselling, communication and active listening skills is essential. The **fpa** has worked with key family planning providers for almost 70 years and has extensive experience in providing training about sexuality and communication to professionals, and in responding to the information needs of the general public as well as providers of family planning and sexual health services. This experience confirms the need for all working in the field of sexual health and family planning to undertake, in addition to appropriate clinical training, experiential training that involves sexuality, exploration of values and attitudes and development of communication skills.

The **fpa** works to support the development of family planning services and provides communication and sexuality training for health and medical professionals (see '**fpa** services', page 213).

Clinical guidelines and audit

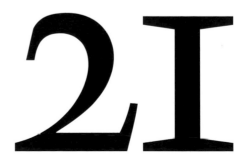

Clinical guidelines are produced to improve the quality of care.

Valid guidelines lead to promotion of cost-effective health care and evidence-based clinical practice which will lead to improvements in clinical outcomes.

Defining clinical guidelines

Clinical guidelines to date have been seen as a variety of things from a voluntary code of practice to a set of prescriptive rules. They have been defined as 'systematically developed statements' to assist in decisions about appropriate care for specific clinical circumstances. Terms such as guidelines, protocols and practice policies are often used interchangeably, often without precise definition.

The NHS Executive defines national clinical guidelines as 'guidelines developed by clinicians and sponsored by the relevant professional body or bodies according to nationally agreed standards. The stronger evidence embodied in them, the more justification there will be for following them.' *(Clinical guidelines – using clinical guidelines to improve patient care within the NHS*, NHS Executive, Good Practice Report, 1996). The term 'local clinical guidelines' refers to 'guidelines which are produced locally and which may or may not be derived from national guidelines'.

Clinical guidelines differ from service guidance which is more directly concerned with issues that can be addressed through the wider commissioning processes and may incorporate components of clinical guidelines. Purchasers and providers need to collaborate in developing and using guidelines, to ensure that both clinical *and* service outcomes are improved.

Developing quality guidelines takes time and resources, will involve systematic review of the evidence base, continuing analysis of health needs and ongoing discussion with professionals and client groups. It is vital that those developing the guidelines are *clear* about the aims and objectives, how they will be measured and evaluated from the start. The process of developing national or local guidelines has important legal implications. As such any development must recognise the need for multi-disciplinary involvement. There is currently no national accreditation system for guidelines, or a central advisory body. However, there are a number of organisations and academic centres set up to provide advice relating to the development, implementation and appraisal of guidelines; for example the Clinical Outcomes Group (COG), the NHS Executive, the Cochrane Collaboration Centre and the Health Care Evaluation Unit (HCEU) at St Georges's Hospital Medical School in London.

Aims of clinical guidelines

Clinical guidelines should aim to be:

▶ VALID: when followed they should lead to the health gains and costs predicted for them
▶ REPRODUCIBLE: given the same evidence and methods another guideline group should produce the same recommendations
▶ RELIABLE: given the same clinical circumstances another health professional should interpret and apply them in the same way
▶ REPRESENTATIVE: all key groups affected should be involved in developing them
▶ APPLICABLE: they should apply to patient populations based upon scientific evidence or best clinical judgment
▶ FLEXIBLE: any exceptions to the recommendations should be identified and it should be indicated how patient preferences are to be taken into account
▶ CLEAR: language must be unambiguous, precise and understandable
▶ METICULOUS: all the evidence and methods used, and participants involved, should be recorded
▶ AUDITED: it should be stated when and how the guidelines are to be reviewed
(Adapted from the NHS Executive Guidance, Good Practice Report, 1996)

There must be close links between clinical guideline development, clinical audit and the monitoring of changes of health outcomes.

Clinical audit

Clinical audit is pivotal in patient care and is the process which brings together the different health care professionals to assess, evaluate and improve the clinical, management and informational aspects of the care of patients/clients in a systematic way to enhance their health and quality of life.

Developing audit involves:

▶ defining standards, criteria, targets or protocols for good practice against which performance can be compared
▶ systematic gathering of objective evidence about performance
▶ comparing results against standards and/or amongst peers
▶ identifying deficiencies and taking action to remedy them
▶ monitoring the effects of action on quality

Clinical guidelines and recommendations for practice in family planning are now being developed by the FFPRHC.

Further reading

Books/reports
Making sense of audit
Irvine D and Irvine S
Radcliffe Medical Press, 1991

Development and implementation of clinical guidelines – Report no 26
RCGP, 1995

Clinical guidelines – what you need to know
Clinical Effectiveness Series
RCN, 1995

Clinical guidelines – using clinical guidelines to improve patient care within the NHS
Mann T
NHS Executive, Department of Health, 1996

Quality assurance guidelines for the cervical screening programme
Report of a Working Party convened by the NHS Cervical Screening Programme
Pritchard J (Chair)
NHSCSP Publications, 1996

Articles

'Developing clinically valid guidelines'
Grimshaw J M, Eccles M P and Russell I T
Journal of Evaluation in Clinical Practice, 1, 1995, 37-48

'Effect of clinical guidelines on medical practice:
a systematic review of rigorous evaluations'
Grimshaw J M and Russell I T
The Lancet, 342, 1993A, 1317-1322

'Achieving health gain through clinical guidelines:
1 – developing scientifically valid guidelines'
Grimshaw J M and Russell I T
Quality in Health Care, 2, 1993B, 243-248

'Achieving health gain through clinical guidelines:
2   ensuring that guidelines change medical practice'
Grimshaw J M and Russell I T
Quality in Health Care, 3, 1994, 45-52

Appendix

Addresses of useful organisations

The fpa in the UK

fpa UK
2-12 Pentonville Road
London N1 9FP
☎ 0171 837 5432 (9am to 5pm)
Contraceptive Education Service Helpline
☎ 0171 837 4044 (9am to 7pm)
www.fpa.org.uk

fpa Cymru
Grace Phillips House
4 Museum Place
Cardiff CF1 3BG
☎ 01222 342766

Bangor Office
Greenhouse, Trevelyan Terrace
Bangor
Gwynedd LL57 1AX
☎ 01248 352176

fpa Northern Ireland
113 University Street
Belfast BT7 1HP
☎ 01232 325488

Derry Office
14 Magazine Street
Derry BT48 6HH
☎ 01504 260016

fpa Scotland
Unit 10, Firhill Business Centre
76 Firhill Road
Glasgow G20 7BA
☎ 0141 576 5088

FP Sales Ltd
Unit 9, Ledgers Close
Nuffield Industrial Centre
Littlemore, Oxford OX4 5JS
☎ 01865 749333

The health promotion agencies of the UK

Health Education Authority
Trevelyan House
30 Great Peter Street
London SW1P 2HW
☎ 0171 222 5300

Health Education Board for Scotland
Woodburn House
Canaan Lane
Edinburgh EH10 4SF
☎ 0131 447 8044

Health Promotion Wales
Ffynnon-las
Ty Glas Avenue
Llanishen, Cardiff CF4 5DZ
☎ 01222 752222

Health Promotion Agency for Northern Ireland
18 Ormeau Avenue
Belfast BT2 8HS
☎ 01232 311611

Medical and nursing organisations

British Medical Association
BMA House
Tavistock Square
London WC1H 9JP
☎ 0171 387 4499

**Committee on Safety of Medicines/
Medicines Control Agency**
Market Towers
1 Nine Elms Lane
London SW8 5NQ
☎ 0171 273 0289

Royal College of General Practitioners
RGCP Centre for Primary Care Research & Epidemiology
Department of General Practice & Primary Care
University of Aberdeen
Foresterhill Health Centre
Aberdeen AB25 2AY
☎ 01224 663131

**Royal College of General Practitioners –
Manchester Research Unit**
Parkway House
Palatine Road
Manchester M22 4DB
☎ 0161 945 6788

Royal College of Nursing
20 Cavendish Square
London W1M 0AB
☎ 0171 409 3333

Practice Nurse Association
RCN
20 Cavendish Square
London W1M 0AB
☎ 0171 647 3867

**Family
planning
organisations**

**Faculty of Family Planning and Reproductive
Health Care (FFPRHC) of the RCOG**
19 Cornwall Terrace
London NW1 4QP
☎ 0171 935 7514

National Association of Nurses for Contraception and Sexual Health (NANCSH)
25 Ledmore Road
Charlton Kings
Cheltenham GL53 8RA
☎ 01242 257751

RCN Family Planning Forum
Royal College of Nursing
20 Cavendish Square
London W1M 0AB
☎ 0171 647 3736

Scottish Society of Family Planning Nurses (SSFPN)
9 William Place
Scone
Perth PH2 6TF

N I Association of Family Planning Nurses
86 Ravenhill Park Road
Belfast BT6 0DG

Margaret Pyke Centre
73 Charlotte Street
London W1P 1LB
☎ 0171 530 3600

Pharmaceutical organisations

Royal Pharmaceutical Society of Great Britain
1 Lambeth High Street
London SE1 7JN
☎ 0171 735 9141

National Pharmaceutical Association
38-42 St Peter's Street
St Albans
Hertfordshire AL1 3NP
☎ 01727 832161

International family planning organisations

International Planned Parenthood Federation (IPPF)
Regent's College
Inner Circle, Regent's Park
London NW1 4NS
☎ 0171 486 0741

Irish FPA
Unity Building
16-17 Lower O'Connell Street
Dublin 1
☎ 00353 878 0366

Natural family planning organisations

Fertility UK
Clitherow House
1 Blythe Mews
Blythe Road
London W14 0NW
☎ 0171 371 1341

Training (in family planning for doctors and nurses)

Faculty of Family Planning and Reproductive Health Care (FFPRHC)
19 Cornwall Terrace
London NW1 4QP
☎ 0171 935 7514 (administration)
☎ 0171 935 7196 (training)

English National Board for Nursing, Midwifery and Health Visiting
Victory House
170 Tottenham Court Road
London W1P 0HA
☎ 0171 388 3131

Welsh National Board for Nursing, Midwifery and Health Visiting
2nd Floor
Colate House
101 St Mary Street
Cardiff CF1 1DX
☎ 01222 261400

National Board for Nursing, Midwifery and Health
Visiting for Scotland
22 Queen Street
Edinburgh EH2 1NT
☎ 0131 226 7371

National Board for Nursing, Midwifery and Health
Visiting for Northern Ireland
RAC House
79 Chichester Street
Belfast BT1 4JR
☎ 01232 238152

**Nurse
prescribing**

Association of Nurse Prescribing
4 Crinan Street
London N1 9SQ
☎ 0171 843 4517

**Clinical
guidelines and
audit**

Clinical Outcomes Group (COG)
Quarry House
Quarry Hill
Leeds LS2 7UE
☎ 0113 2545972

UK Cochrane Centre
Summertown Pavillion
Middleway
Oxford OX2 7LG
☎ 01865 516 300

Cochrane Fertility Regulation Review Group (FRRG)
Leiden University, Medical Centre
Gynaecology and Reproductive Medicine
Department of Clinical Epidemiology
K6P – 076
PO Box 9600
NL 2300, RC Leiden
Netherlands

Young people

Brook Advisory Centres
(Head Office)
165 Gray's Inn Road
London WC1X 8UD
☎ 0171 713 9000

Youth Access
1A Taylor's Yard
67 Alderbrook Road
London SW12 8AD
☎ 0181 772 9900

Sex education

fpa (see 'fpa services', page 213)

Sex Education Forum
National Children's Bureau
8 Wakley Street
London EC1V 7QE
☎ 0171 843 6000

Abortion

Birth Control Trust
2-12 Pentonville Road
London N1 9FP
☎ 0171 278 4809

Unplanned pregnancy

British Pregnancy Advisory Service (BPAS)
Austy Manor
Wootton Warren, Solihull
West Midlands B95 6BX
☎ 01564 793225
☎ 0345 304030 for information

Marie Stopes House
108 Whitfield Street
London W1P 6BE
☎ 0171 388 0662
☎ 0800 716390 for information on local centres

Relationships

RELATE – England
Herbert Gray College
Little Church Street
Rugby
Warwickshire CV21 3AP
☎ 01788 573241
For local centres see telephone or local help directory

RELATE – NI
76 Dublin Road
Belfast BT2 7HP
☎ 01232 323454

Marriage Counselling Scotland
105 Hanover Street
Edinburgh EH2 1DJ
☎ 0131 225 5006

Jewish Marriage Council
23 Ravenshurst Avenue
London NW4 4EE
☎ 0181 203 6311

**Marriage Care
(previously Catholic Marriage Advisory Centre)**
Clitherow House
1 Blythe Mews
Blythe Road
London W14 0NW
☎ 0171 371 1341

**ACCORD
(previously Catholic Marriage Advisory Centre – NI)**
76 Lisburn Road
Belfast BT9 6AF
☎ 01232 491919

Infertility	**ISSUE (The National Fertility Association)** 114 Lichfield Street Walsall West Midlands WS1 1SZ ☎ 01922 722888
	CHILD Charter House 43 St Leonard's Road Bexhill-on-Sea East Sussex TN40 1JA ☎ 01424 732361
	Human Fertilisation and Embryology Authority (HFEA) Paxton House 30 Artillery Lane London E1 7LS ☎ 0171 377 5077
Sexuality issues	**The Albany Trust** The Art of Health and Yoga Centre 280 Balham High Road London SW17 7AL ☎ 0181 767 1827
Lesbian and gay support	**Gay Switchboard** BM Switchboard London WC1N 3XX ☎ 0171 837 7324
General women's health	**Women's Health** 52 Featherstone Street London EC1Y 8RT ☎ 0171 251 6580
One parent families	**National Council for One Parent Families** 255 Kentish Town Road London NW5 2LX ☎ 0171 267 1361

Cancer organisations

CancerBACUP
3 Bath Place
Rivington Street
London EC2A 3JR
☎ 0171 696 9003

Women's Nationwide Cancer Control Campaign (WNCCC)
Suna House
128-130 Curtain Road
London EC2 3AR
☎ 0171 729 2229

Breast Cancer Care
Kiln House
210 New Kings Road
London SW6 4NZ
☎ 0171 384 2984

STIs including HIV/AIDS

For details about NHS genitourinary medicine (GUM) services, contact the **fpa** Contraceptive Education Service Helpline on
☎ 0171 837 4044 (Monday to Friday, 9am to 7pm)

National AIDS Trust
New City Cloisters
188-196 Old Street
London EC1V 9FR
☎ 0171 814 6767

National AIDS Helpline
☎ 0800 567123 (24 hour freephone)

Terrence Higgins Trust
BM AIDS
London WC1N 3XX
☎ 0171 242 1010 (helpline)
☎ 0171 831 0330 (administration)

**Pregnancy
organisations**

Maternity Alliance
5th Floor
45 Beech Street
London EC2P 2LX
☎ 0171 588 8582

National Childbirth Trust
Alexandra House
Oldham Terrace
London W3 6NH
☎ 0181 992 8637

Miscarriage Association
Clayton Hospital
Northgate, Wakefield
West Yorkshire WF1 8JS
☎ 01924 200799

SATFA (Support after Termination for Fetal Abnormality)
73-75 Charlotte Street
London W1P 1LB
☎ 0171 631 0285

SANDS (Stillbirth and Neonatal Death Society)
28 Portland Place
London W1N 4DE
☎ 0171 436 7940

PMS support

PREMSOC
PO Box 102
London SE1 7ES

National Association for PMS (NAPS)
PO Box 72
Sevenoaks
Kent TN13 1QX
☎ 01732 760012

Menopause support

The British Menopause Society (for professionals)
36 West Street
Marlow
Buckinghamshire SO7 2NB
☎ 01628 890199

The Amarant Centre (charity)
Churchill Clinic
80 Lambeth Road
London SE1 7PW
☎ 0171 401 3855

The Amarant Trust
11-13 Charterhouse Building
London EC1M 7AN
☎ Helpline 01293 413000

National Osteoporosis Society
PO Box 10
Radstock
Bath BA3 3YB
☎ 01761 471771

Psychosexual problems

Institute of Psychosexual Medicine
11 Chandos Street
London W1M 9DE
☎ 0171 580 0631

Association of Sexual and Marital Therapists
Box 62
Sheffield S10 3TS

The Association of Psychosexual Nursing
PO Box 2762
London W1A 5HQ

Further general reading

See also the end of each chapter for further specific reading.

Contraception and family planning

▶ ***Contraception and sexuality in health and disease***
Sapire, K Esther
(UK edition revised and updated by T Belfield and J Guillebaud)
McGraw Hill, 1990
NOTE: *out of print, useful for comprehensive data and references up to 1990*

▶ ***RCN guidelines for domiciliary family planning***
RCN, 1993

▶ ***Contraception – your questions answered***
Guillebaud, J
2nd edn, Churchill Livingstone, 1993, revised 1994
(new edition due mid-1999)

▶ ***Handbook of family planning and reproductive health care***
Loudon N, Glasier A and Gebbie A (eds)
3rd edn, Churchill Livingstone, 1995

▶ ***The economics of family planning services – a report prepared for the Contraceptive Alliance***
McGuire A and Hughes D
fpa, 1995

▶ ***Managing family planning in general practice***
Rowlands S
Radcliffe Medical Press, 1997

▶ *Contraceptive choices: supporting effective use
of methods*
Walsh J, Lythgoe H and Peckham S
CES, **fpa**, 1996

▶ *Improving access to quality care in family planning:
medical eligibility criteria for contraceptive use*
WHO, Geneva, 1996

▶ *Directory of hormonal contraceptives (international)*
Kleinman R L (ed)
3rd edn, IPPF, 1996

**Sexually
transmitted
infections**

▶ *ABC of sexually transmitted diseases*
Adler M W
4th edn, BMJ Publishing, 1998

▶ *ABC of AIDS*
Adler M W
4th edn, BMJ Publishing, 1997

▶ *A general practitioner's guide to genitourinary medicine
and sexual health*
Sonnex C
Cambridge University Press, 1996

▶ *Sexually transmitted infections nursing care and
management*
Steadman T
Stanley Thornes, 1998

**Sexual health/
sexuality**

▶ *Human sexuality and its problems*
Bancroft J
2nd edn, Churchill Livingstone, 1989

▶ *Contraceptive care – meeting individual needs*
Montford H and Skrine R (eds)
Chapman and Hall, 1993

▶ *Women's sexual health*
Andrews G (ed)
Baillière Tindall, 1996

▶ *Sexual health promotion in general practice*
Curtis H, Hoolaghan T and Jewitt C (eds)
Radcliffe Medical Press, 1995

▶ *Sexual history-taking in general practice*
Jewitt C
The HIV Project, 1995

Infertility

▶ *Infertility – guidelines for practice prepared by Fertility Committee of RCOG*
1992
(being revised)

Hormone replacement therapy

▶ *Hormone replacement therapy – your questions answered*
Whitehead M and Godfree V
Churchill Livingstone, 1992
new edition due Autumn 1999

Premenstrual syndrome

▶ *PMS – the complete guide to treatment options*
Hayman S
Piatkus, 1996

General

▶ *Women's Health*
McPherson A (ed)
4th edn, Oxford University Press, 1997

▶ *Counselling in medical settings*
East P
Open University Press, 1995

fpa services

Contraceptive Education Service (CES)

Contraceptive
Education
Service

Would you like more information about family planning?

CES provides a range of services to health professionals and the public across the UK.

Leaflets on contraception

Special CES leaflets on all 13 methods of contraception are available for the primary health care team and family planning professionals to use with their clients. All leaflets are consumer-tested and written to plain English standards using expert medical advice. The leaflets, which are regularly updated, are free from local health promotion units, and larger orders can be placed directly with the **fpa** at a low cost. Call 01865 719418 for details.

CES Helpline

The nationwide CES Helpline runs Monday to Friday and provides:

► confidential information and advice to the public and professionals on all aspects of contraception, sexual and reproductive health
► details of local family planning services and GUM clinics anywhere in the UK

► **fpa** UK ☎ 0171 837 4044 (9am to 7pm)
► **fpa** Cymru ☎ 01222 342766 (9am to 5pm)
► **fpa** Scotland ☎ 0141 576 5088 (9am to 5pm)
► **fpa** Northern Ireland ☎ 01232 325488 (9am to 5pm)

Information services

The *Contraceptive Education Bulletin* is a quarterly journal for professionals on family planning and reproductive health. CES factsheets are also available on a range of topics. Visitors are welcome to use the CES library and information centre at the **fpa**'s London address, which carries the latest medical, legal and statistical information.

CES is run in England in partnership with the Health Education Authority, in Northern Ireland with the Health Promotion Agency for Northern Ireland, in Wales with Health Promotion Wales, and in Scotland with the Health Education Board for Scotland.

Education and training

Do you need more support or training in delivering your sexual health and family planning services?

The **fpa** has pioneered training and consultancy on sexuality, sex education, personal relationships and communication for professionals working in health, medical, education and community settings. The service, which is highly respected and renowned throughout the UK, is provided through our centres in London, Wales (Cardiff and Bangor), Northern Ireland (Belfast and Derry) and Scotland (Glasgow).

Publications for professionals

Do you need practical, accessible, informative resources to support you in your work?

The **fpa** has developed a unique range of publications for health and other professionals on sexuality, sex education and contraception. In addition to the reports included on suggested reading lists within this handbook, the **fpa** publishes training manuals, classroom resources, handbooks and reference guides. For full details of **fpa** and other publications, please contact the **fpa**'s mail order service, **fpa direct**, PO Box 1078, East Oxford DO, Oxfordshire OX4 5JE, ☎ 01865 719418.

Publications for the general public

An accessible range of **fpa** publications is available for the public at low cost. Bulk orders can be supplied to professionals. Contact the **fpa**'s mail order service, **fpa direct**, PO Box 1078, East Oxford DO, Oxfordshire OX4 5JE, ☎ 01865 719418.

The **fpa**'s popular *Sexual Health Series* provides many of the answers that patients seek from busy health professionals. All booklets are evidence-based and contain useful contacts and further reading sections. Discounts available for bulk purchase.

Infertility Tests and Treatment (1998)

Explains the reasons for difficulty in conceiving, when to seek help, the various treatments that are available and advice on how to obtain treatment and select a specialist clinic. This accurate and authoritative booklet addresses the complex issues raised by infertility in an accessible, friendly way.

The menopause (1996)

A booklet explaining what happens during the menopause, how women can seek advice and what they can do to help themselves.

Planning a pregnancy (1996)

Information and advice for women who want to get pregnant.

Publications for young people

The **fpa**'s popular booklets for young people are all available in bundles of 50 for just £12 including p&p.

LOVE S.T.I.NGS (1999)

In brilliant comic strip style, this booklet raises and answers young people's questions about STIs – their symptoms and long-term effects, how they are treated, and how they can be avoided. Above all, it presents a reassuring picture of the sexual health clinic and the importance of a check-up if there is any reason to think you could have an STI.

Is Everybody Doing It? Your Guide to Contraception (1996)

Deals with peer pressure, the issues involved in starting a sexual relationship, going to a family planning clinic, different contraceptive methods and STIs. For 13 to 17 year olds.

4Girls: a below-the-bra guide to the female body (1997)
This colourful booklet uses simple text and humorous illustrations to give girls aged 12 to 16 the facts they want to know about physical changes and sexual development.

4Boys: a below-the-belt-guide to the male body (1996)
Information on testicular self-examination, contraception, STIs and safer sex. Full colour, highly illustrated booklet for young men aged 13 to 16.

Periods: what you need to know (1996)
This colourful booklet prepares young girls aged 9 to 12 for menstruation – why girls and women have periods, what happens and how to deal with it.

FP Sales Ltd

FP Sales Ltd, the commercial arm of the **fpa**, provides a medical supplies service designed to meet the needs of those in general practice and NHS family planning, reproductive and sexual health clinics. Because of its connection with the **fpa**, FP Sales offers a wide range of family planning products and educational items from leading manufacturers as well as a comprehensive range of medical supplies. Each year all the profits of FP Sales Ltd are covenanted to furthering the work of the **fpa**.

For further details or a catalogue, contact
FP Sales Ltd
Unit 9, Ledgers Close
Nuffield Industrial Centre
Littlemore, Oxford OX4 5JS
☎ 01865 749333